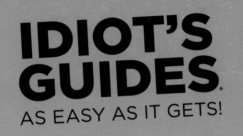

IDIOT'S GUIDES
AS EASY AS IT GETS!

Hairstyles

by Kylee Bond

ALPHA

A member of Penguin Group (USA) Inc.

ALPHA BOOKS

Published by Penguin Group (USA) Inc.

Penguin Group (USA) Inc., 375 Hudson Street, New York, New York 10014, USA · Penguin Group (Canada), 90 Eglinton Avenue East, Suite 700, Toronto, Ontario M4P 2Y3, Canada (a division of Pearson Penguin Canada Inc.) · Penguin Books Ltd., 80 Strand, London WC2R 0RL, England · Penguin Ireland, 25 St. Stephen's Green, Dublin 2, Ireland (a division of Penguin Books Ltd.) · Penguin Group (Australia), 250 Camberwell Road, Camberwell, Victoria 3124, Australia (a division of Pearson Australia Group Pty. Ltd.) · Penguin Books India Pvt. Ltd., 11 Community Centre, Panchsheel Park, New Delhi—110 017, India · Penguin Group (NZ), 67 Apollo Drive, Rosedale, North Shore, Auckland 1311, New Zealand (a division of Pearson New Zealand Ltd.) · Penguin Books (South Africa) (Pty.) Ltd., 24 Sturdee Avenue, Rosebank, Johannesburg 2196, South Africa · Penguin Books Ltd., Registered Offices: 80 Strand, London WC2R 0RL, England

International Standard Book Number: 978-1-61564-704-0
Library of Congress Catalog Card Number: 2014943481

16   15   14   8   7   6   5   4   3   2   1

Interpretation of the printing code: The rightmost number of the first series of numbers is the year of the book's printing; the rightmost number of the second series of numbers is the number of the book's printing. For example, a printing code of 14-1 shows that the first printing occurred in 2014.

Note: This publication contains the opinions and ideas of its author. It is intended to provide helpful and informative material on the subject matter covered. It is sold with the understanding that the author and publisher are not engaged in rendering professional services in the book. If the reader requires personal assistance or advice, a competent professional should be consulted. The author and publisher specifically disclaim any responsibility for any liability, loss, or risk, personal or otherwise, which is incurred as a consequence, directly or indirectly, of the use and application of any of the contents of this book.

Most Alpha books are available at special quantity discounts for bulk purchases for sales promotions, premiums, fund-raising, or educational use. Special books, or book excerpts, can also be created to fit specific needs. For details, write: Special Markets, Alpha Books, 375 Hudson Street, New York, NY 10014.

Trademarks: All terms mentioned in this book that are known to be or are suspected of being trademarks or service marks have been appropriately capitalized. Alpha Books and Penguin Group (USA) Inc. cannot attest to the accuracy of this information. Use of a term in this book should not be regarded as affecting the validity of any trademark or service mark.

Publisher: *Mike Sanders*

Executive Managing Editor: *Billy Fields*

Development Editorial Supervisor: *Christy Wagner*

Senior Designer: *Becky Batchelor*

Senior Production Editor: *Janette Lynn*

Indexer: *Johnna VanHoose Dinse*

Layout Technician: *Brian Massey*

Proofreader: *Monica Stone*

Photography: *Becky Batchelor Photography*

Contents

TOOLS OF THE TRADE 3

Styling Products.................... 4

Styling Tools 10

Styling Aids 14

HAIRSTYLING BASICS........ 17

Adding Volume 18

Taming Frizz 20

Getting Shiny Hair 22

STYLES FOR SHORT HAIR....25

Sleek and Straight..................26

Twisted..........................30

Short Hair Blowout 34

Tousled Texture 38

Polished Pompadour 42

Sleek Look 46

Curly Girl 50

Side Swept 54

Short and Sassy Pony.............58

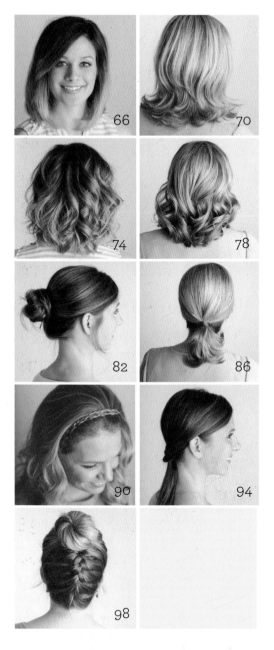

STYLES FOR MEDIUM-LENGTH HAIR 65

Basic Blowout 66

Flipped Out 70

Beach Waves 74

Polished Coils 78

Undone Bun. 82

Party Pony 86

Braided Headband 90

Inside-Out Pony. 94

Upside-Down Braided Knot. 98

STYLES FOR LONG HAIR....103

Basic Braid......................104

French Braid 108

Prairie Braid....................112

Inchworm Braid 118

Braided Bun....................122

Fishtail.........................126

Bombshell Curls.................130

Mermaid Waves 134

Top Knot 138

High Roller......................142

Polished Pony 146

Knot Your Basic Bun.............150

Crown and Glory 154

Festival Braided Knot.............158

Bear Claw Ponytail 164

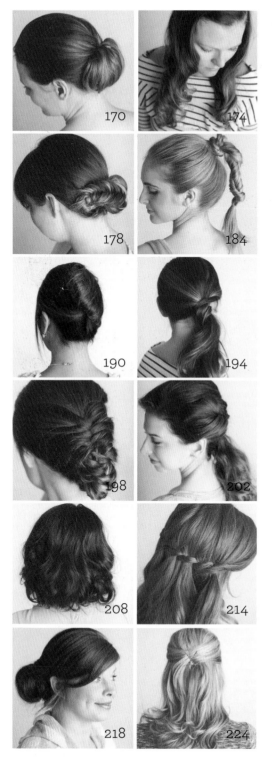

STYLES FOR SPECIAL OCCASIONS. 169

Simple Chignon. 170

Retro Waves. 174

Fishtail Bun 178

Twisted Pony. 184

French Twist 190

Side-Swept Pony. 194

Broken Fishbone 198

Half Twist 202

Faux Bob 208

Waterfall Braid 214

Side Bun 218

Half Up. 224

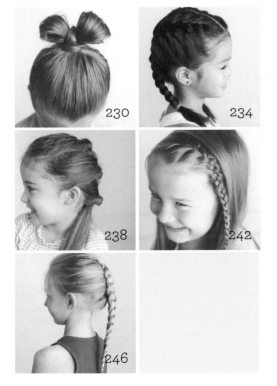

230
234
238
242
246

SUPER STYLES FOR GIRLS. 229

Hair Bow 230

Double French Braid 234

Twisted Sister 238

Braided Fringe 242

Inside-Out French Braid 246

Glossary 252

Index 260

Introduction

I'm instantly taken back to my first trip to the salon with my mother. Maybe you have a similar memory of that occasion with your own mom. I can remember the entire atmosphere: the smells, the sounds, the products, the stylist. But most of all, I remember my mother's demeanor when we left the salon. She seemed happy and confident with her new look. She also seemed to have an extra pep in her step that afternoon. Something about that day resonated with me, and I couldn't wait to go back to get my hair styled to feel just as beautiful as my mother did. Looking back now, as someone in the role of hairstylist, it's my goal to make everyone who sits in my chair or reads this book look and feel their absolute best.

Even if you've never picked up a curling iron, teasing comb, or bobby pin, I assure you that you *can* create a variety of hairstyles, whatever your hair length, with the help of this book. In it, I explain the best ways to prep your hair before you begin a style and explain what tools and styling products to use and when. Then the fun begins, as I walk you, step by step, through each of the 50 styles and show you how to create salon-worthy finished looks at home—complete with tips on fun ways to accessorize your new 'do.

Learning to style your own hair shouldn't be frustrating—it should be rewarding! Take your time and follow the easy, how-to steps laid out in *Idiot's Guides: Hairstyles*. It may take you a few tries to master the basic steps, but once you learn the essentials, you'll be styling your hair into that party-perfect ponytail or pompadour with no effort at all. (If you find an area you're unsure of, simply turn back to the hairstyling basics pages or to the glossary for additional assistance.)

One of the most confusing aspects of hairstyling is knowing what type of product to use on your hair and how and when to apply it. Product manufacturers produce collections of items specific to every hair type that benefit each texture, so that's a good place to start. It's best to work with what you have naturally and gently coax it to behave how you want it to. In addition to product distribution and usage, certain styling techniques also aid in creating specific looks. I cover all of this and more in the following pages.

When you're ready for a bit more of a challenge, I've included formal styles that take you from birthday party to red carpet, as well as some looks for the little ladies in your life. None of these are styles to be intimidated by! Simply follow the text instructions and the helpful photos, and soon you'll see that these styles are really quite doable!

Read this book cover to cover, or pick and choose the parts that interest you most. However you use it, you're sure to gain a wide variety of techniques and skills to build your hairstyling knowledge with the help of this guide. Everything I've included has been helpful to me along the way, and I hope the same is true for you as you discover how fun and rewarding it can be to style your own hair. You'll save money, gain tons of confidence in your abilities to style your own hair, and look and feel beautiful—as if you've just stepped out of the salon!

Acknowledgments

I'd like to extend an enormous thank you to my team at Alpha Books for all their enthusiasm, hard work, and help making this book as fabulous as it can possibly be: my editor Christy Wagner, book designer/photographer Becky Batchelor, and managing editor Billy Fields. Thanks to Christie Wright and Mary Landwer for their helpful assistance in making the hairstyles come to life. Also, thanks to Tess Payton for her mad makeup skills and making our models look their personal best. Thank you to all the beautiful models—Alicia Mummert, Brittany Case, Carly Grant, Christie Wright, Heather Stafford, Jenni Davis, Jessica Kelly, Josie Sanders, Jourdyn Berry, Julie and Kennedy Williams, Kirsten Becker, Kristi and Mia Johnson, Marian Bender, Mary Landwer, Monica Johnson, Mya Fields, Shelby Dock, and Sophia Batchelor—for taking time out of your busy schedules to help create the images for this book. Next, I owe an enormous amount of gratitude to my husband, Ryan, for holding down the fort while I was hard at work trying to make this book come to life, but most of all for always believing in me. My friends and family ... you all know who you are. It's a great comfort to know that I have an awesome support system and that you all have cheered me on throughout this incredible journey, especially Ronny Douglas, Judy Bond, and Christy Rushton. As they say, "it takes a village," and I have an amazing one behind me. A huge thanks to my mother, Marcia, for encouraging me to always do my best and believing I could truly do whatever I set my heart to. In addition, thank you to my clients and the readers of this book for allowing me to live my dream as a professional hairstylist. I appreciate each and every one of you and realize this all would not be possible without you. It's truly an honor to be able to make people look and feel their best.

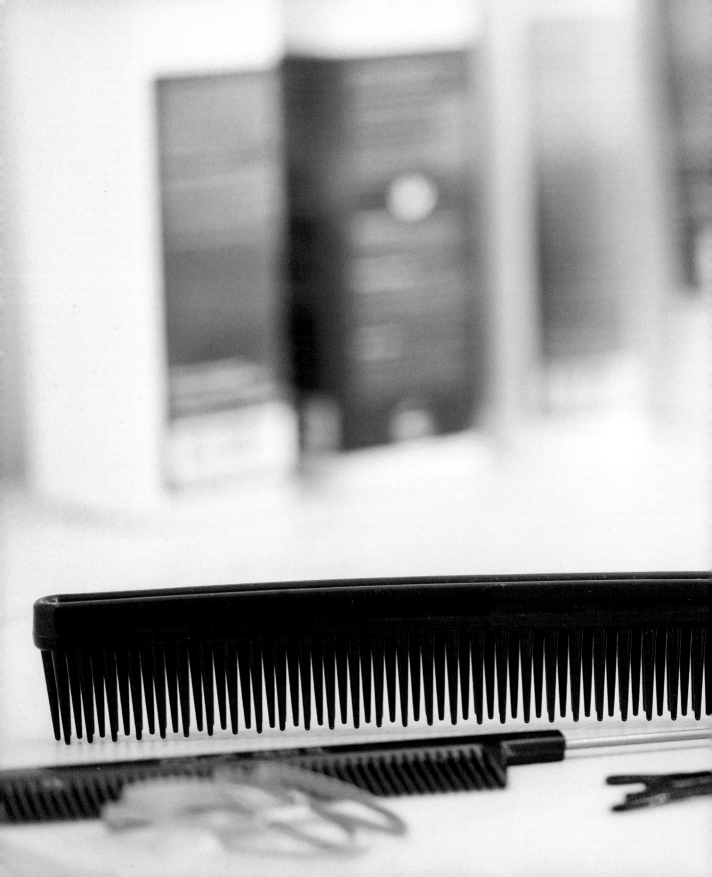

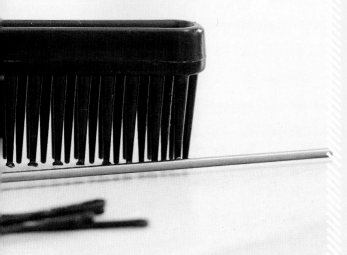

TOOLS
of the Trade

Hair styling tools and gadgets come and go, but it's important to learn the basic, classic styling tools; their purpose; and how to correctly use them. In this first part, you meet the styling products, tools, and aids recommended for the hairstyles in this book. Some you might already have; some might be new to you. But rest assured; I share tips and tricks on how and when to use each.

If you've ever seen a fantastic hairstyle and wondered how the wearer achieved that look, you can stop wondering after reading this section. The tool descriptions clearly explain what each tool and product does so you can achieve the style you desire. These are everyday styling helpers you can find at your local beauty supply store and are easy to manage with a few simple techniques and a little practice.

Styling Products

With so many styling products available at your hair salon, on drugstore and big-box store shelves, and online, trying to decide what shampoo, conditioner, or other styling products are best for your hair can be confusing. Rather than purchasing a generic, one-size-fits-all product for convenience, it's really better to take some time to learn about the various products available so you can use what's best for your specific hair.

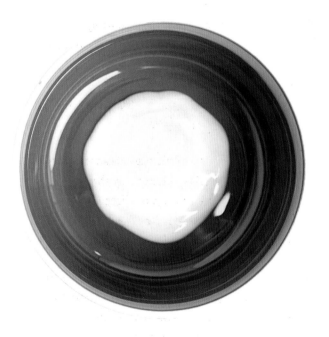

When you're shopping for shampoos, it's best to steer clear of any product that contains alcohol or harsh chemicals.

Shampoo

Shampoo manufacturers produce cleaners for myriad types and textures of hair. Here are a few types you might see:

Volumizing shampoo   This lightweight shampoo is meant to give limp locks some lift. It's usually (or should be) clear in color and should give your hair a weightless feel. This purifier shouldn't strip your hair of its natural oils.

Thickening shampoo   This shampoo is best for those whose hair is thinning or who have very fine hair to begin with. It normally contains an exfoliating ingredient to give your strands the best possible foundation for growth. Half of the reason hair doesn't grow—other than genetics—is follicle asphyxiation, meaning your follicles are smothered and, therefore, stop growing. The thickening shampoo helps clear away what's smothering your follicles so your hair can grow again.

Hydrating shampoo   This cleanser is normally a bit heavier and made for dry or dull hair. If you have fine hair, you'll most likely want to avoid hydrating or moisturizing shampoos because they could weigh down your hair. Medium to thick and coarse hair types benefit most from this cleanser.

Repairing shampoo   This shampoo shifts your hair into repair mode after your mane has been abused with heat or harsh chemicals. It also helps reduce breakage.

Dry shampoo   This shampoo is every girl's best friend and a quick and easy hairstyle extender. By using this oil-absorber, you can get away with a 2- or 3-day-old style. You also can add texture to your hair by applying dry shampoo to your roots and teasing with a teasing comb. This is great for formal styles as well.

Conditioner

After shampooing your hair clean, conditioner is one of the first styling products you put back in your hair. Conditioners have a variety of uses and types:

Volumizing conditioner   This weightless formula is meant to soften your tresses without leaving behind any residue that might weigh down your 'do. Fine to medium hair types benefit from a lightweight cream conditioner.

Hydrating conditioner   If you have a curly coif or are prone to frizz, this is the conditioner for you. A hydrating conditioner containing aloe or olive oil can naturally help your hair revive itself.

Use a hydrating conditioner during the dry winter months to ward off static.

Repairing conditioner   This rejuvenating product often contains a type of protein or keratin treatment to help strengthen weak or damaged hair. If you frequently color your hair or use hot tools in it regularly, you should use this type of conditioner at least once a week.

Thickening conditioner   This conditioner is meant to be used alongside thickening shampoo and adds natural volume to limp or lifeless stands. This booster softens and separates your strands without weighing them down.

Leave-in conditioner   This conditioner comes in either a cream or a spray. Most leave-in treatments contain a moisture-retention ingredient as well as something to help protect your hair. In addition, these revitalizers can come in different levels of moisture depending on your hair type. Most also help with shine.

Dry conditioner   You can use this product to hydrate your hair from the middle of your strands to the ends; it absorbs oil as it works. Some contain sunflower oil or argan oil for additional moisture.

Styling

This category is often the largest—and also the most confusing! The lifters, lotions, powders, and other potions in this section all have specific uses and can smooth, tame, boost, or add bounce to your hairstyle:

Root lifter   This root booster gives you lift at the root or your hair or in your crown area. Opt for a root lifter that's not full of stickiness, but one that leaves your hair soft and touchable.

Sculpting lotion   This light-hold gel formula gives hair hold without weighing it down. It's best to use before you curl your hair or to add longevity to your style.

Styling foam   Also known as mousse, this multitasking product can be used to add volume not only to your roots, but also to the ends of your hair while providing a light hold. Mousse, or styling foam, tames and forms your hair but doesn't leave it crunchy and dry. All hair types and textures benefits from this product.

Firm-hold gel   This gel is built to set your hair with maximum hold. You might see formal styles and up-dos call for this product before blow-drying to ensure the style lasts all night. If you have curly hair that's somewhat defiant, you might try using this gel for some better control.

Thickening lotion   This plumper, designed to cover each of your strands to make them fuller, is best for very fine hair that needs more body. It can double as a light-hold product as well.

Volumizing powder   Sprinkle this fairy dust-looking product on your roots for added fullness. Some even reactivate throughout the day with a little heat and friction from your fingers. This gives you a tousled, voluminous look.

Curl cream   This multipurpose product defines your curls while also providing a light hold—without weighing down your locks like other products can do. You can layer curl cream with a light- or firm-hold gel for maximum hold in your style.

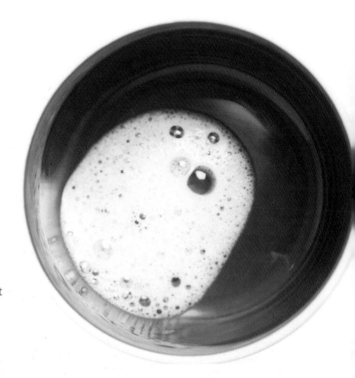

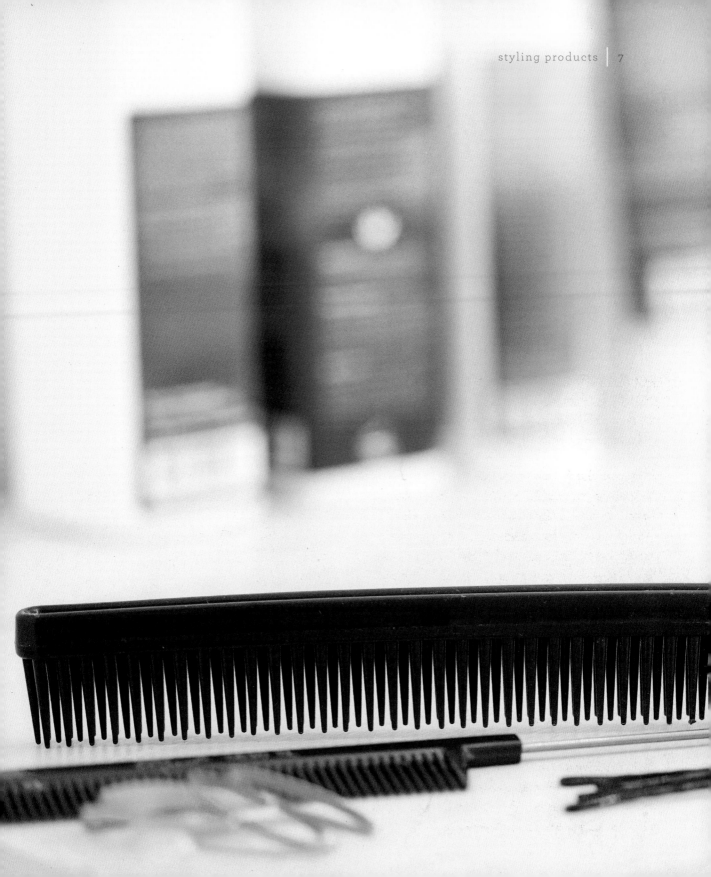

Sea-salt spray   This blend, which you typically spray on the ends of your hair, assists in creating a natural wave look. Those with naturally wavy or curly hair can achieve soft waves by using this mist; straight strands can get texture and a touch of bend.

Volumizing hairspray   A hairspray that promotes volume with a firm hold. It usually has stronger hold to help hold and amplify hair for a voluminous look.

Working hairspray   A working hairspray is brushable and provides moveable hold. This spray should be heavy enough to hold the style, but not give you a stiff look or feel.

More recently, lighter-weight working hairsprays are dry. The dry sprays provide hold without the stickiness that often accompanies wet sprays.

Maximum-hold hairspray   This hairspray usually includes an antihumectant ingredient that protects your hair from the environment to prolong your style. Some can feel stiff when in your hair; however, other modern, heavy-hold sprays contain lighter ingredients that won't weigh down your hair. Max-hold sprays are typically used in formal styles or ones you don't want to move ... at all.

Antifrizz serum   A product that combats frizz by surrounding your hair strands with a protective, moisturizing coating. Depending on the type of serum, it can be used wet or dry and works best to combat frizz and tame unruly hair. In some cases, it can even reduce the time your hair takes to dry.

Antihumectant serum   A styling product that protects your hair from the environment. It blocks moisture, preventing frizz, and can help smooth your hair and tame flyaways.

Argan oil   This oil, produced from kernels from a tree grown in Morocco, contains vitamins and essential fatty acids beneficial for your hair. It's ideal if your hair is in distress or needs moisture. As it absorbs into your hair, it hydrates and repairs. It can be used on wet or dry locks.

Moisturizing serum   This product—be it argan oil, an antifrizz serum, or any kind of serum that contains moisturizing ingredients—is used to soften and relax hair.

Shine spray   Used mostly as a finishing product, this mist is designed to enhance shine and bring life to dull hair. If you don't wash your hair every day, using this spray in addition to the dry conditioner could revive the ends of your hair. You also might like using this spray before you gently comb through your curls.

Smoothing serum   This product, which could be considered a moisturizing serum, typically contains an antifrizz or antihumectant property to coax wavy, coarse, or curly hair smooth and straight. Many also now contain protectants to help prevent future damage.

Thermal protectant   If you frequently use hot tools, you also should frequently use this product. Thermal protectant is normally sold as a spray or cream and contains essential oils to hydrate your hair. In addition, it helps protect your hair from humidity and contains beneficial antioxidants and proteins.

Spray wax   A new delivery of an old favorite, this wax has a light to medium hold that's meant to add a touch of texture and grit to hair. Fine to medium hair types will benefit from this tress plumper.

Defining paste   This is a lightweight finishing product can be used to softly mold your hair. Shorter hairstyles can really reap the benefits of this paste; applying a small amount throughout your hair adds texture.

Texture putty   Similar to defining paste, this putty gives you a strong yet workable hold. Texture putty works best for shaping shorter styles.

Many are transparent and can be used on all hair types, but if the putty is light in color, it's best to use it on lighter-colored hair.

Pomade   This light-hold finishing product defines your strands and adds polish and shine.

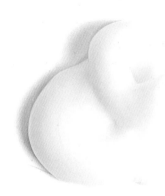

Styling Tools

You don't need a lot of specialized tools or equipment to style your hair, but some basics will come in handy for many looks. Here are some commonly used hairstyling tools you might want to have:

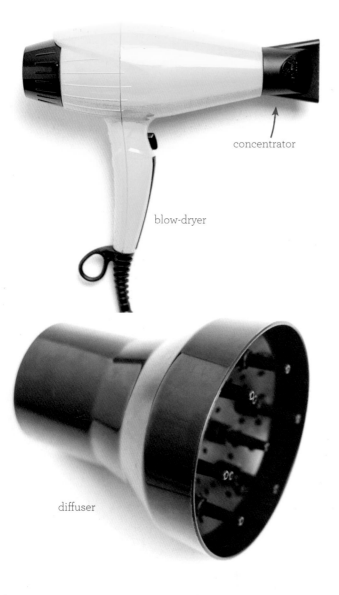

concentrator

blow-dryer

diffuser

Blow-dryer   This indispensable tool blows hot air or cool air at various speeds. A blow-dryer's main purpose is to dry wet hair, but you also can use it to help form your hair into a specific style, such as a blowout. For smooth and shiny hair, a blow-dryer, a round brush, and a small amount of product are all you need—no flat iron required!

Concentrator   This device fits on the end of a blow-dryer and concentrates and directs air and heat flow through so you can dry your hair smoothly. Using a concentrator on your blow-dryer means you can get smoother and more polished hair without the use of a straightening iron.

Diffuser   This attachment fits on the end of your blow-dryer and is designed to enhance your curls by diffusing the air and heat widely and evenly. It also reduces frizz when drying curly hair.

curling iron   flat iron

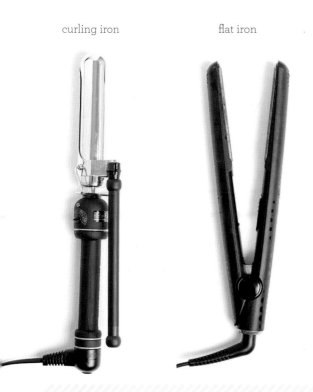

Curling iron A curling iron is a handheld tool with a barrel on one end that heats up. You coil your hair around the hot barrel, close the clamp to keep your hair against the barrel, hold for a few seconds, and unclamp for curly locks. Multiple barrel sizes are available, ranging from $^3/_8$ inch (1cm) to 2 inches (5cm). The larger the barrel, the larger your curls.

Flat iron A flat iron, or straightening iron, is another handheld tool that uses heat to style your hair. This tool has two ceramic plates that close together, sandwiching your hair in between, to smooth and flatten your hair. Flat irons can get extremely hot, reaching temperatures upward of 400°F (205°C).

Other irons or curling helpers you might find include *curling wands, three-barrel curling irons,* and *crimping irons.*

A curling wand is basically a clampless curling iron. This heated rod is great for getting mermaid waves.

Three-barrel curling irons have three barrels—typically two on the bottom and one on the top. Pressing your hair between the barrels creates soft, uniform waves.

Crimping irons kink your hair into sharp, chevron or zigzag waves. This look was popular in the 1980s but is making a comeback on runways and costume parties everywhere.

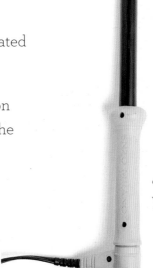

curling wand

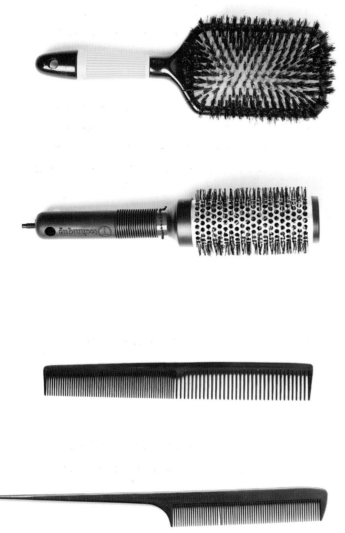

Paddle brush   This large, flat brush is used to detangle and help reduce drying time when blow-drying. The bristles are designed to be gentle on wet and dry strands. It can even give you a slight scalp massage when you brush through your hair thoroughly.

Round brush   This brush will soon become your favorite. It's essential for smoothing, taming, and curling your hair. Opt for a vented version if you can find one. Many sizes of round brushes are available to yield different styles. A smaller round brush produces a curly or wavier look on the middle and ends of your hair. A larger size mainly smooths your hair and adds a slight bend at the ends.

All-purpose comb   This general comb has many uses, hence the name. It's best to have one that's heat resistant so you can use it to guide and keep your hair smooth while you use heat-producing styling tools. A good general comb can also be used to mold hair into up-dos.

Rattail comb   This comb has small teeth on one end and a straight, pointy pick on the other end. The pointy end is helpful for precisely sectioning and parting your hair before styling.

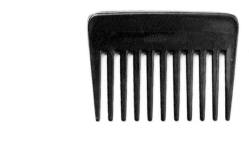

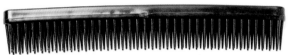

Wide-tooth comb   The teeth on this comb are spaced a bit wider apart than on other types of combs. This helps you gently work through tangles.

Teasing comb   This comb contains three rows of teeth and is used to backcomb your hair to create more volume. Don't use just any comb to tease your hair; a teasing comb is vital for creating volume without damaging your hair.

Teasing brushes and *vent brushes* are two other types of brushes you might want to try.

Teasing brushes usually contain nylon and boar bristles and are used similarly to teasing combs to add volume or texture.

Vent brushes have slots, or vents, in the body of the brush, between the bristles. When you use a vent brush as you blow-dry your hair, air flows through these vents and around your hair, enabling you to dry it faster.

Styling Aids

Styling tools and products are two categories of hairstyle helpers, but these styling aids are often crucial to creating—and keeping—your look:

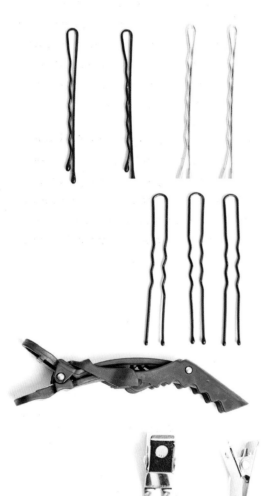

Bobby pins These little pins hold your hairstyle in place, and they're an especially essential part of an up-do style. Most standard-size bobby pins are about 2 or 3 inches (5 to 7.5cm) long. (Larger and smaller sizes are also sold.) Bobby pins come in a variety of colors to blend in to many hair colors.

Hairpins These U-shape pins are similar to bobby pins but are meant to secure your locks without disrupting the flow of the hairstyle. Whereas a bobby pin offers firm hold, hairpins have a very loose and natural hold. This is due to their design—both legs of hairpins are smooth, and they're separated a bit more than the legs of bobby pins. Hairpins also come in different lengths and colors.

Clips Many sizes, shapes, and types of hair clips are available, but most often in this book, *clip* refers to a sturdy pinching clip with grips on one side to hold hair in place. You can find these clips at your beauty supply store.

Duckbill clips These silver metal clips are approximately 2½ inches (5cm) long and have two prongs. The duckbill clip is commonly used to hold and set curls after they've been curled with a curling iron.

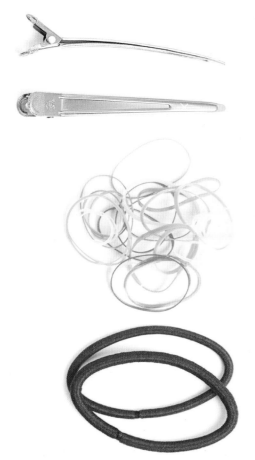

Long metal clips These long, flat, and metal clips range from 2 to 4 inches (5 to 10cm) long. This type of clip is commonly used to hold curls or mold hairstyles without leaving any creases like a duckbill clip might.

Elastic bands The clear version of these rubber bands, often no larger than $1/2$ to $3/4$ inch (1.25 to 2cm) in diameter, are commonly used in up-styles and formal hairdos. Because they're clear, they camouflage into your hair, so no one but you knows they're there. Colored elastic bands are also available and are perfect for little girls. These add a pop of color to the end of a braid or around ponytails. You can match every outfit with these fun colors.

Stretchy ponytail holders These larger, stretchy bands contain a coating over the elastic or rubber band so they don't pull or break your hair when you're putting them in or taking them out. These bands come in different sizes to suit a variety of hair thickness. They're great for securing ponytails for maximum hold if the clear elastic isn't strong enough.

Two other styling aids you might find helpful when creating hairstyles at home are *fabric hairbands* and *sock bun sponges*.

Fabric hair bands (Emi-Jay is one brand) are a modern, decorative version of a hair tie for when you want a quick and easy splash of color in your hair.

Sock bun sponges help you form the perfect bun. These doughnut-shape sponges enable you to pull your ponytail through the center hole and then pin your hair around the doughnut to create a full, round bun. If you have trouble forming a voluminous bun with just your hair alone, try a sock bun sponge. They're available in different colors and sizes.

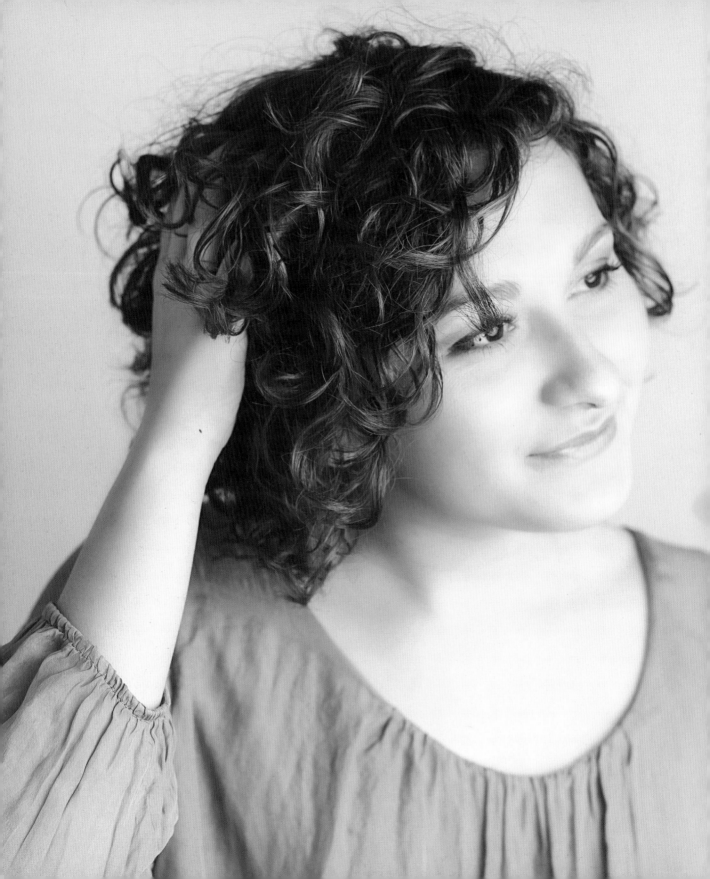

Hairstyling
BASICS

Just like you can't build a house without any carpentry or construction skills, you shouldn't expect to create perfect 'dos without first learning the basics of hairstyling. In this section, I share the building blocks necessary for the foundation of many of the styles in this book, including how to add volume, tame frizz, and achieve shiny locks.

It's easy to overlook the importance of prepping your hair before beginning a style. How you prep your hair determines how it behaves in the finished hairstyle. If you do a poor job prepping, you can forget that pretty style you'd hoped to attain. Prep also depends on what type of hair you have. If you have curly hair, for example, you'll likely use heavy, moisturizing products to get your strands ready to style, while someone with straight, fine hair will use a cocktail of volume builders to amplify their style. No matter your hair type, texture, or length, I show you the best way to treat your tresses.

Adding Volume

If your locks are more limp and lifeless than you'd like them to be, you can create volume in your hair. Let's look at how to build body and create fullness for different types of hair.

Fine Hair

If you have fine hair, whether it's straight or wavy, yours requires the most manipulation to create volume. Thoroughly towel dry your hair. Apply a thickening serum, and comb it through your hair from the roots to the tips. Next, add a root-lifting spray (either a foam or a spray form should work) to your scalp in your crown area. Lastly, add a styling foam or a mousse through the middle lengths and ends of your hair for voluminous hold.

Medium-Thick Hair

If your hair isn't fine but isn't thick, you'll still have a bit of work to do to add volume. If your hair is straight, follow the directions for adding volume to fine hair, but skip the thickening serum. Your medium-thick hair has a bit more density and doesn't need it.

If your hair is wavy, you'll use some different products. When your hair is damp, add a root lifter to your scalp in your crown area.

You also can add a light moisturizing serum for moisture and control of your waves. The serum helps alleviate frizz when you're adding volume. Then finish with an application of mousse to the middle and ends of your hair.

Thick Hair

Thick hair requires the most moisture. With straight hair, you might be able to skip a heavy moisturizing serum and opt for a lighter one. However, the volumizing process is the same. When your hair is damp, apply a moisturizing serum. This will penetrate your hair shafts and retain moisture. Next, you'll seal in the moisture but still create volume. Use a mixture of sculpting gel and shine spray to help with moisture retention and hold. Lastly, you can add a mousse or a bit more gel to the ends of your hair for maximum volume.

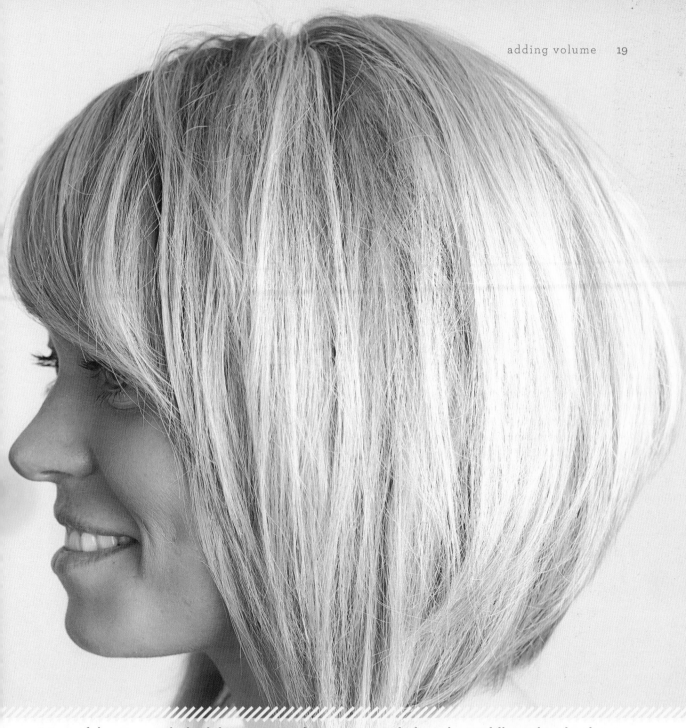

Most of the time with thick hair, extra volume isn't needed on the middle and ends of your hair, so you can skip the mousse or more gel if you feel you have enough thickness already.

Taming Frizz

Frizz can ruin an otherwise lovely look, and to make matters worse, it can be one of the hardest hairstyle problems to fix. Taming frizz has to do primarily with the condition your hair is in. The most important consideration is the moisture level of your hair.

Fine Hair

If you have fine hair and frizz, it's most likely due to breakage around your hairline or new, baby hairs growing in in that area.

To tame frizz in fine hair, you can first use a light moisturizing serum to tend to the lack of moisture if there is one. Then you can apply a moisture sealant the middle and ends of your hair to lock in moisture.

If absolutely necessary, you also can use an antifrizz serum after applying the moisture sealant but before you blow-dry your hair. If your hair still looks as if it has flyaways, use a bit of defining paste to push down the flyaways after your hair is dry.

Medium-Thick and Thick Hair

Medium-thick hair that's wavy and thick hair that's curly need the most moisture and are typically the most prone to frizz.

If you have either of these types of hair, first use a moisturizing serum when your hair is damp; apply it throughout the middle and ends of your hair. Next, use an antifrizz serum on the middle and ends of your hair to tame the frizz and act as an antihumectant barrier.

Dry your hair with a blow-dryer and use a paddle brush to pull your hair smooth when drying. Be sure to blow-dry from the roots to the ends, pushing your hair cuticle downward to avoid creating additional frizz.

If you tend to dry your hair upside down, be sure to still blow your hair from the roots to the ends. That's one of the most common mistakes people make when drying their hair and trying to remove frizz.

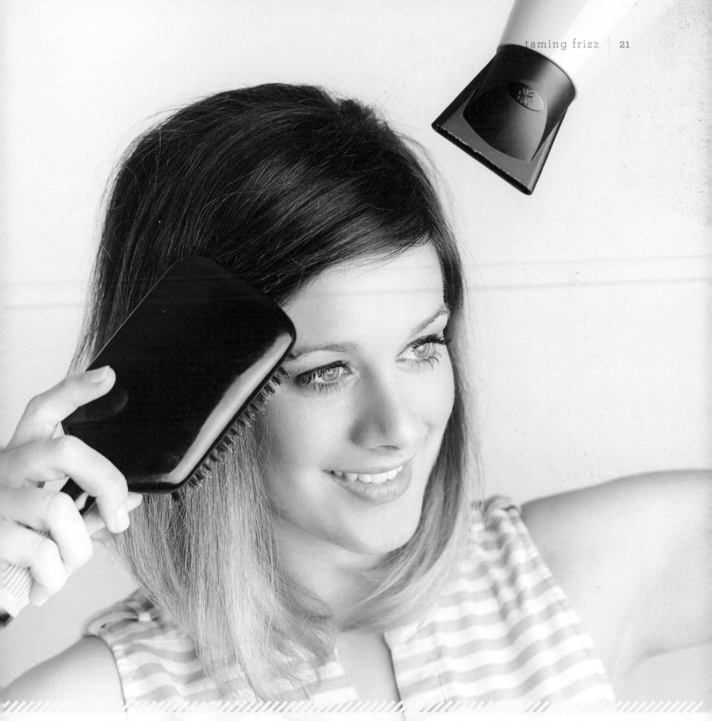

When working with fine hair, be extremely careful not to oversaturate it with heavy products or ones that use fillers, such as silicone or heavy waxes. I recommend layering products—and using the right products—for best results. Using high-quality products is also key.

Getting Shiny Hair

The main reason hair isn't shiny is often because it's unhealthy due to lack of moisture or it has been damaged somehow. Hot styling tools and chemical-laden hair colors and other products can strip your hair of its natural moisture. And believe it or not, washing your hair every day isn't necessarily a good thing. The repeated washing removes your hair's natural oils that are necessary to keep your hair in its optimal condition. With the combination of repeated washing, the stripping of its natural oils, and the use of hot tools and chemicals, it's no wonder your hair can get dull.

The first step back to silky, shiny strands is to evaluate your shampoo and conditioner. Use a moisturizing or repairing shampoo and conditioning system to help your hair get back to its natural healthy state. Using a moisturizing serum or protectant on your hair when it's damp before you blow-dry can replenish some of the moisture you've lost, too.

You might want to forgo your blow-dryer if your hair is in a fragile condition. If you're trying to restore your hair's health and have to use some type of hot tool, it's better to skip the blow-dryer and just use the hot tool. If you blow-dry your hair when its damaged and then use a hot tool right after that, you increase the risk of damage.

In addition to maintaining your hair's optimal health, you can add a shine mist or polishing serum to the ends of your hair after your style is complete. With either product, use it in moderation on the middle and ends of your hair.

I hope all these tips help you better understand a few fundamentals of styling. One of the most important steps of a style is how you prep your hair. If the prepping is done incorrectly, you most likely won't achieve the result you were hoping for. Remember these helpful hints, and you'll increase your chances for fabulous hair.

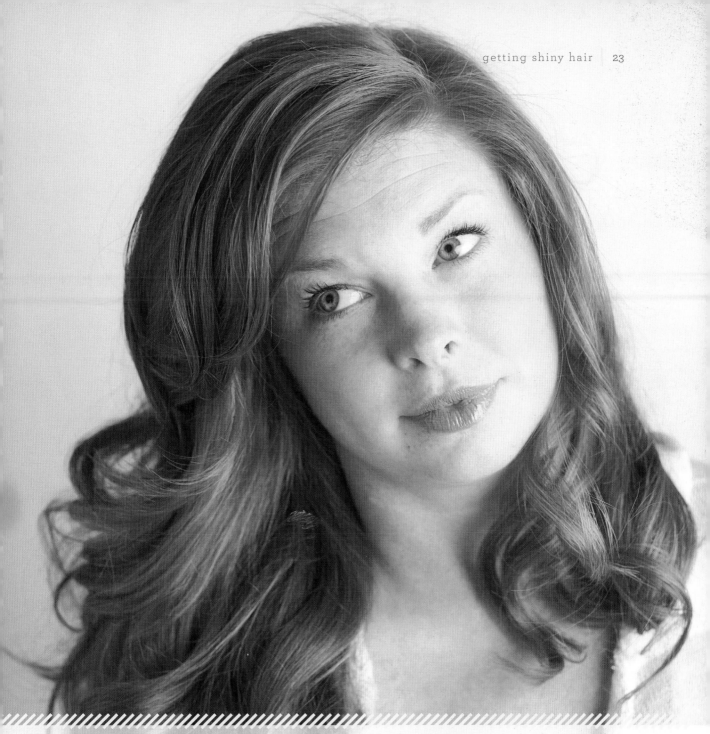

Look at ingredient lists to see what's actually in the products you use on your hair, and be sure they don't contain fillers. You want pure ingredients for optimal hair health. Heavy silicones or waxes can zap the shine right out of your hair.

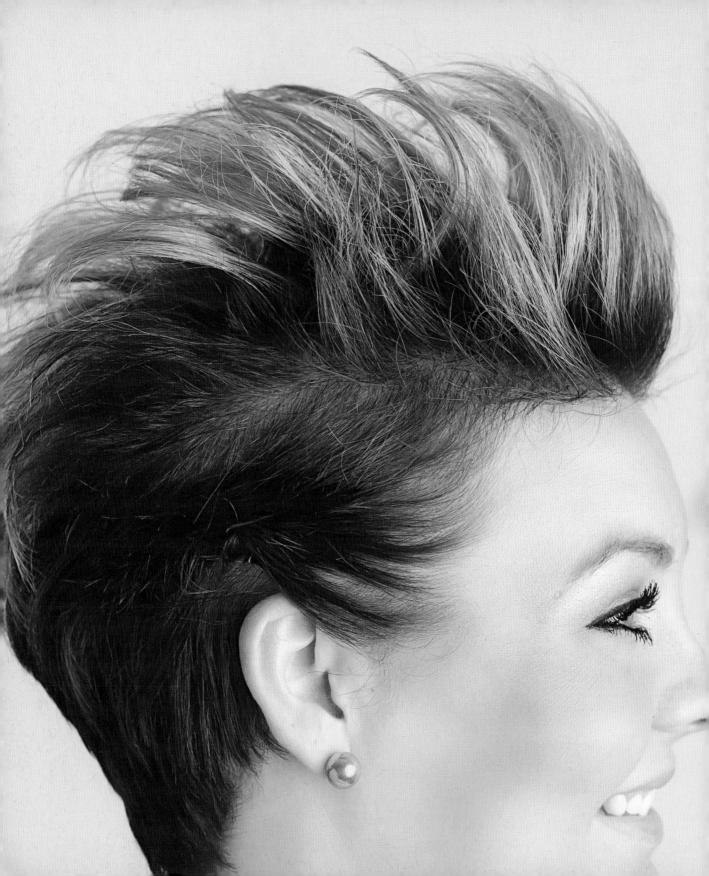

Styles for
SHORT
Hair

If you want quick and easy-to-care-for hair, a short style can be the solution. However, it's all too common for women to cut their hair short and then not take the time to style it to its full potential.

It can be fun and even exciting to cut your hair to a short crop cut—but don't stop there! Take pride in your short strands and wear them well! In the following pages, you learn to style your short cut to bring out the best in your mane and create versatility and adaptability in your hairstyle.

Sleek and Straight

This style should be a staple in every woman's hairstyle arsenal. All types of hair can get the sleek and straight look by adding the correct products, tools, and skills. If you have straight hair, you can use a flat iron mostly for taming and smoothing flyaway hairs; if you have wavy or curly hair, you'll need to straighten and tame your curls to get the polished and silky look. Straightened hair is very versatile. You can wear this look to a business meeting or out to coffee with friends, or spice it up for an evening out with your special someone.

TOOLS NEEDED

blow-dryer	heat-resistant comb
clips	iron guard spray
concentrator	light- to medium-hold hairspray
flat iron	
glossing drops (optional)	paddle brush

PREPPING YOUR HAIR | Thoroughly

towel dry your hair before applying any product. If you have fine or straight hair, use a combination of root lifter and volumizing mousse for additional movement. If you have medium to thicker strands with texture (wavy or curly), tame and condition your hair with a moisturizing oil and then add an antihumectant serum to coat your hair and keep frizz at bay. Wavy- and curly haired ladies also might want to add a volumizing spray at the roots to boost volume on the top while still having smooth strands.

1

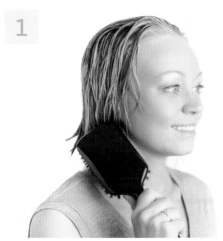

Start with thoroughly towel-dried hair. Apply product as necessary depending on your hair type, and gently brush through your hair with a paddle brush.

2

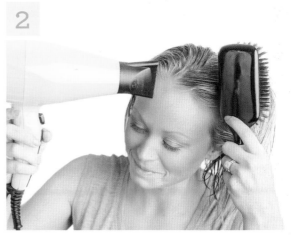

Using the paddle brush and your blow-dryer fitted with a concentrator, blow-dry your hair from the roots to the ends in opposite directions, creating soft volume, until your hair is dry.

3

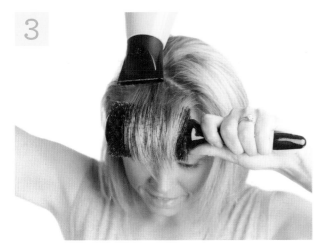

If you have bangs, or fringe, blow-dry that area until your cowlicks are relaxed, if you have any. It's best to tame cowlicks while your hair is wet. When it's dry, hair is more difficult to mold.

4

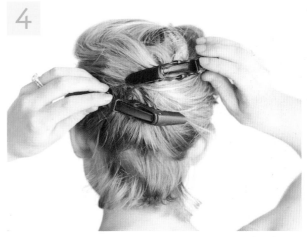

When your hair is completely dry, separate out a section of hair at the nape of your neck about 1 inch (2.5cm) up from your hairline, and pull the rest up and out of the way and secure it with clips.

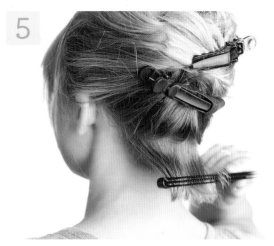

Spray your hair with an iron guard spray to prevent damage. Then, working in the section of loose hair, separate a subsection about 2 inches (5cm) wide. Place a heat-resistant comb under that subsection, lifting it about 45 degrees away from where it naturally falls.

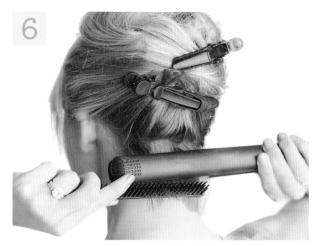

Place the flat iron as close to the base of your scalp as you can for maximum sleekness. Close the iron, and slowly glide it down your hair, slightly tilting the iron under at the end of your hair. Repeat on another 2-inch (5cm) subsection, and continue until you've straightened the whole section at the nape of your neck.

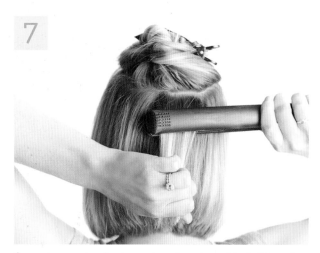

Separate another horizontal section about 1 inch (2.5cm) wide above the one you just straightened, and repeat steps 5 and 6. Continue with this method until you reach the crown of your head.

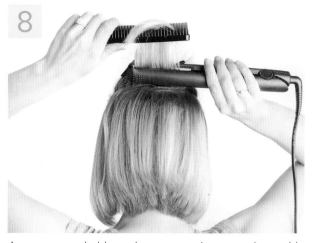

At your crown, hold your hair at a 90-degree angle to add volume and body. You want your hair to be sleek and straight but not lifeless against your scalp. To do this, insert the comb at 90 degrees under the hair at your crown, and place the flat iron at the base of your scalp. Glide slowly to the ends of your hair in a fluid motion. This motion should take about 4 to 6 seconds, depending on the length of your hair.

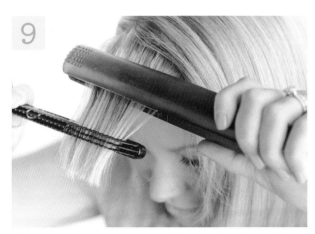

9

If you have bangs, you can now flat iron them. Insert the comb under your bangs at about a 45-degree angle—just enough to lift them off your forehead—and smooth them with the flat iron.

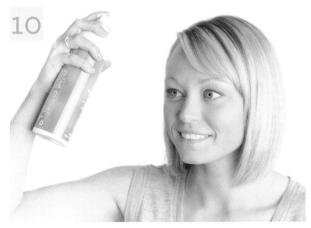

10

Now finish with a light- to medium-hold hairspray. If you have wavy or curly hair, you might want to add some additional humidity resistance with glossing drops.

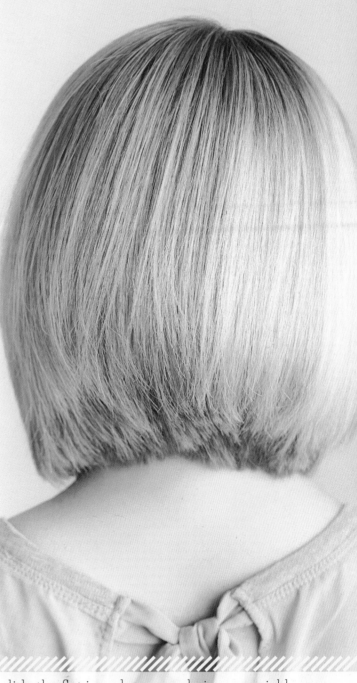

It's a common misconception that you need to glide the flat iron down your hair very quickly multiple times to achieve smooth, shiny tresses. To use this technique correctly, it's best to move slowly and steadily down your hair just one time. You may go a second time if needed for stubborn, coarse pieces.

Twisted

This fun style works best with short hair that's between the lengths of a pixie cut and a short, inverted bob, and wavy and curly hair will benefit the most from this style. You even can let your natural texture shine with a little enhancement from products made to define and shine, such as a pomade or molding paste. This is as easy as it gets if you're looking for a low-maintenance 'do.

TOOLS NEEDED

blow-dryer
concentrator
defining paste
diffuser (optional)

PREPPING YOUR HAIR | If you have fine strands, reach for volumizers with hold, like a volumizing mousse. You also can layer a powder lifter for extra volume before blow-drying if you'd like. Medium to thicker tresses need a little less volume and more hold. If you have medium-length hair, you might want to use a mousse as well. If you have coarse and thick locks, first use a moisturizing serum to control frizz, and follow that with a cocktail of a light-hold gel or mousse over top.

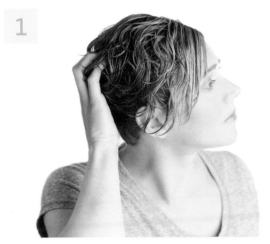

Start with damp hair. Apply the appropriate product for your type of hair.

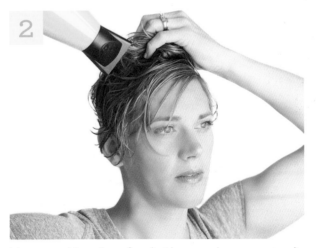

Using your blow-dryer, fitted with a concentrator, on medium heat and low flow, gently tousle strands as you blow out some of the moisture. If your hair doesn't have a whole lot of texture to begin with, you can enhance its body by using a diffuser on your blow-dryer. Blow-dry your hair until it's about 80 percent dry for curly hair, and between 90 and 95 percent dry for wavy or less-textured hair.

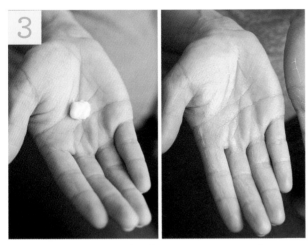

Pump a small amount of defining paste in your palm, about $^3/_4$ inch (2cm) in diameter. Rub your palms together until the product is almost transparent on your hands and all you see is a slight sheen.

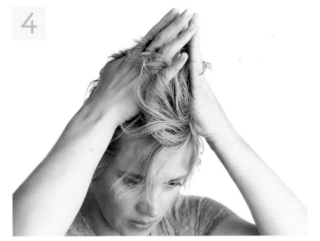

Push the heels of your hands through the base of your hair and work up to the tips, thoroughly coating your hair with the proper amount of product.

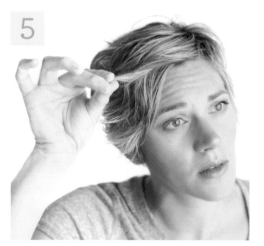

For added definition, use the product leftover on your fingertips to define and twist the pieces you want to add texture to.

If you have bangs, one fun adaptation to this style is to twist your bangs, starting at the base of your hair and continuing to the end. Secure that piece with a bobby pin or hairpin, and voilà! You've got textured bangs!

Or you can add a subtle jeweled headband for daytime wear or a glitzed-up version for evening wear.

If you have finer hair, you might want to add a dry spray wax to your hair for extra movement and height.

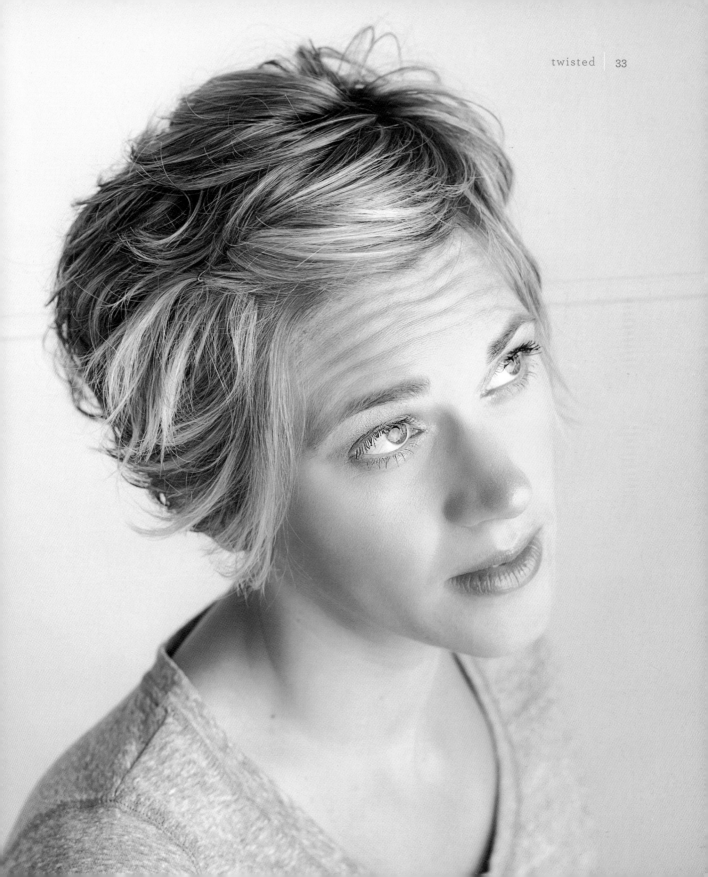

Short Hair Blowout

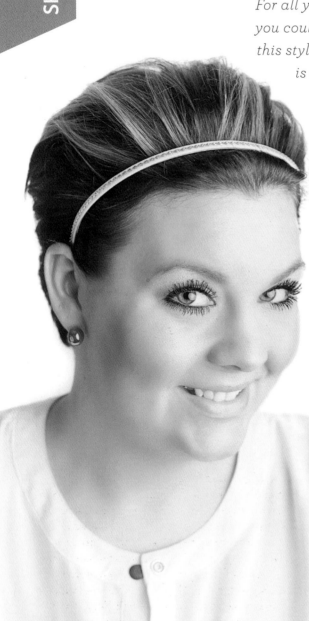

For all you lovely ladies with short hair who didn't think you could achieve a polished, easy, everyday look at home, this style is going to prove that thought wrong. The blowout is one of the most versatile hairstyles around. Wash and style your hair Monday morning with a fresh blowout, and by midweek, add simple adjustments to transform your blowout into multiple 'dos to take you from your children's bus stop to your anniversary dinner date. All hair types can enjoy this style.

TOOLS NEEDED

blow-dryer

clips

concentrator

defining paste

medium-hold hairspray

paddle brush

round brush

wide-tooth comb

PREPPING YOUR HAIR | All hair

should be thoroughly towel dried before applying product. Those with fine hair should use a cocktail of root lifter and volumizing mousse for some extra bounce. If you have medium to thick strands, add volume and hold with a light-hold gel or styling glaze and combat any frizz with a smoothing serum. Those with thick, coarse, or curly tresses, focus first on softening with a moisturizing serum and then add mousse or gel for hold and shine.

1

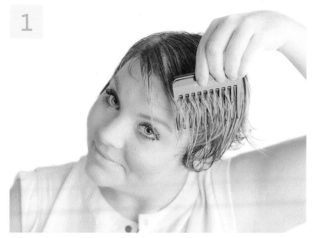

Start with thoroughly towel-dried hair. Apply product as necessary, depending on the type of hair you have, and gently comb through your hair with a paddle brush or wide-tooth comb to avoid tangles.

2

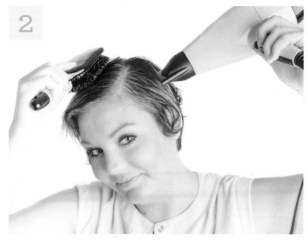

Add a concentrator on the end of your blow-dryer for correct tension and heat flow. Then use the paddle brush and blow-dryer to dry your hair from the roots to the ends in opposite directions to create volume.

3

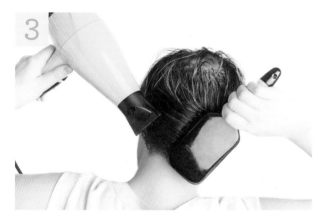

As you're moving to the back of your head and pushing your paddle brush back and forth, blow all your hair to one side and let it naturally shape around your head. After you've gotten out most of the moisture on that side, switch to the other side and continue pushing your hair to the opposite side to let it naturally have a little bend. Continue drying your hair until it's about 80 percent dry.

4

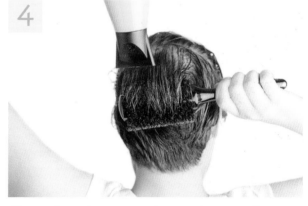

Clip up all your hair except a horizontal section of hair about 2 inches (5cm) wide at the nape of your neck (or as high as you have to go to get enough hair to wrap around the brush). Insert the round brush at a 45-degree angle underneath the subsection, and with a concentrator on your blow-dryer and using medium heat and firm tension, gently glide from the base of your hair to the ends. When you reach the ends, spin the round brush a couple times with the heat still on it to enhance the curl at the end. Repeat with another section of hair about 2 inches (5cm) wide above the section you just completed until you reach your crown.

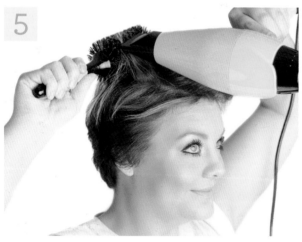

At your crown, hold the round brush under your hair at a 90-degree angle from your scalp to create maximum volume. Use the brush and blow-dryer as you did for the rest of your hair to create polished volume at your crown.

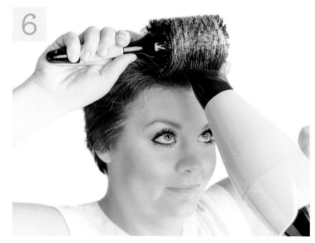

Along your front hairline, direct your hair at 90 degrees up and back, away from the face. Tease your hairline to add volume around your face if you have fine hair.

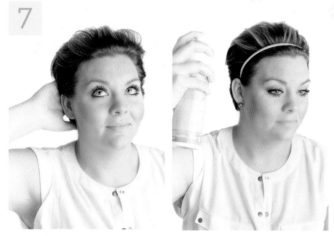

Use defining paste to smooth the sides, and finish with a medium-hold hairspray. For a little extra sparkle, add a pretty headband to dress up this style.

If you have full bangs, you can use the round brush in a forward motion, let it cool for a few seconds on the brush, and then drop your hair. This should ensure your bangs lay nicely. If you have a side-swept fringe, it's best to round brush forward first with good tension and then slightly tilt your brush to the side, with the concentrator firmly pressed against the brush. You can blow your hair all the way to the ends and drop without cooling.

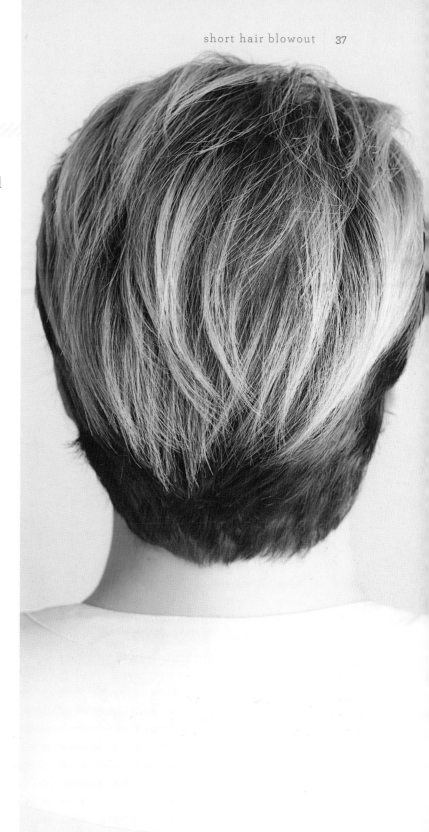

If you have tapered or shorter hair at the back of your head, walk the round brush down the back of your head. (You might need a smaller round brush for this.) When your hair is about 80 percent dry, clip the longer hair up and out of the way. Starting just above your occipital bone, the bony bulge you feel just above the nape of your neck, push the round brush firmly against your head. Then place the concentrator on the round brush, and roll your hair from the roots to the ends with the heat on it. This technique helps short hair look just as polished in the back as in the front.

Tousled Texture

You lucky ladies with natural texture will love this style that tames yet enhances your curly or wavy locks. It's amazing what the right kind and amount of product can do for your style. You can go from drab *to* fab *in about 10 minutes with an easy new go-to hairdo. Although this is a simple style, you can easily dress it up for special events—it's so versatile. If you have fine and/or straight strands, you might want to try another style if you think you don't have enough natural texture to create this look.*

TOOLS NEEDED

antifrizz/moisturizing serum

antihumectant hairspray

blow-dryer

bobby pins (optional)

curl cream

defining paste

diffuser

PREPPING YOUR HAIR |

For this style, you want your hair to be slightly damp to start. You can towel dry it, but it should still have some moisture in it before you apply product.

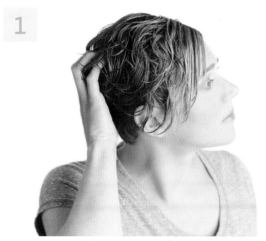

Start with damp hair. Squeeze a small amount of antifrizz or moisturizing serum, about $1/4$ to $3/4$ inch (.5 to 2cm), into your palms and rub into palms. Apply the serum to your hair, from your ears downward. (To avoid an oily look, don't apply to your root area.)

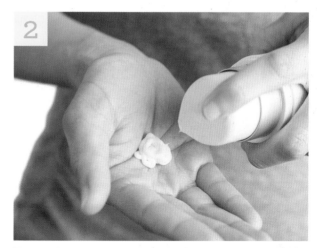

To enhance your natural texture, apply a dollop of curl cream about 1 inch (2.5cm) in diameter evenly throughout your hair; still avoid your scalp.

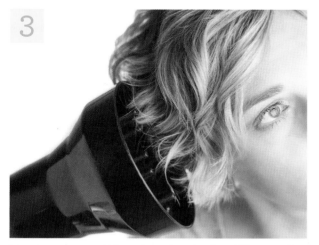

Now you can use a blow-dryer, fitted with a diffuser, on low heat to enhance your curl but minimize frizz. Dry your hair until it's about 75 percent dry if you have curly hair. If your hair is wavy, dry to about 90 percent.

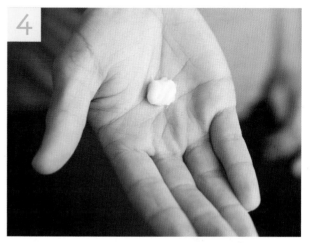

When your hair is dried to the desired amount, it's time to apply some defining paste. Squeeze a dollop about $7/8$ inch (2.25cm) in diameter into the palm of your hand.

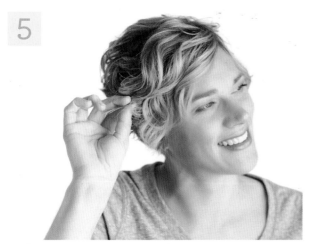

Now get creative! Pick and choose individual sections of hair that are frizzy or unruly, and glide down them with your fingers that have the paste on them.

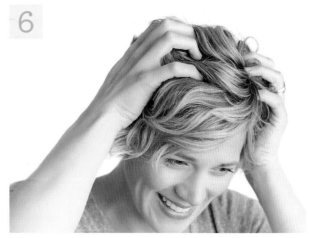

After you've applied paste to individual sections, you can go back through and add another drop of paste and scrunch it into your hair for additional bounce.

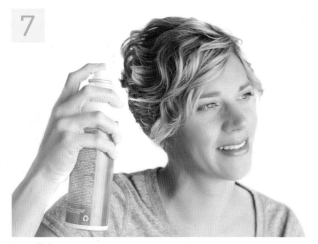

To finish, spray your hair with an antihumectant hairspray to keep your style intact and frizz free.

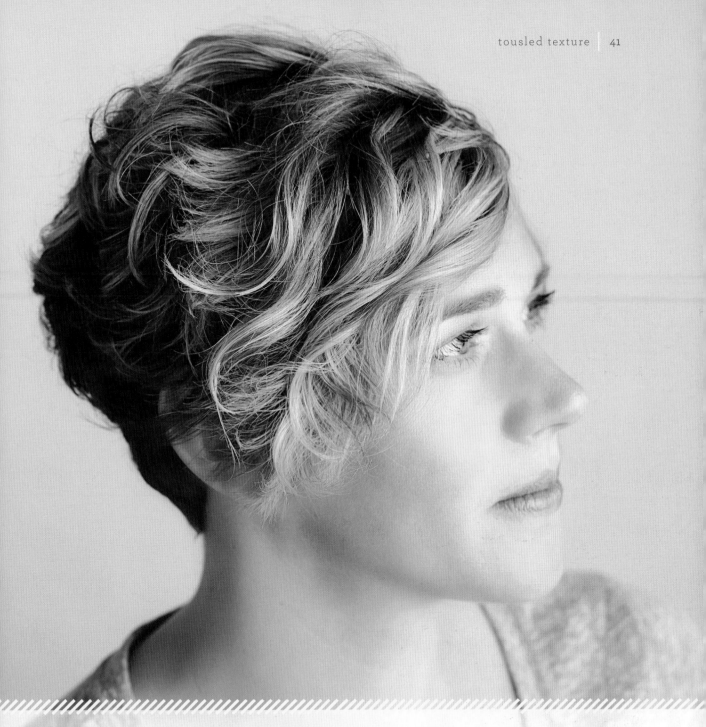

Curly hair tends to shrink about 2 to 2^1/$_2$ inches (5 to 6.5cm) when it's dry, so the fringe area commonly hangs forward into the eyes. If you want, pin your bangs back away from your face with bobby pins, going with the natural flow of your wave or curl and gently pinning them back to one side.

Polished Pompadour

The pompadour is a 1940s hairstyle that's making a comeback. This trendy look is a contemporary way for you to style your hair away from your face—and also have a little hair attitude! This style is perfect for a night out dancing with friends or a special event, but probably not one for the office or casual days. In fact, the edgier version of this style has recently been gracing Hollywood's red carpets. All textures of hair can attempt this style, even different lengths. Those with natural texture will need a bit more prestyle prepping.

TOOLS NEEDED

bobby pins

medium- to firm-hold hairspray

molding paste (optional)

paddle brush

rattail or teasing comb

shine spray (optional)

working hairspray

PREPPING YOUR HAIR | Before you
even begin to dry your hair for style, it's important to use a volumizing shampoo and conditioner first. This allows your hair to have maximum volume as you tease it into the pompadour. Apply a volumizing product—either a root spray or volumizing mousse—close to the roots of your clean, dry hair. Then blow-dry your hair while lifting up on the roots to get maximum volume.

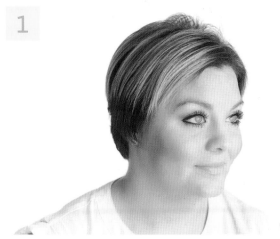

1 Start with dry hair that's been prepped with a working hairspray for hold. (If your hair is too soft and fine, it won't hold the style.)

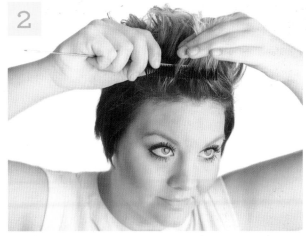

2 Use a rattail comb or a teasing comb to separate a section out of hair in the front part of your hair. This should be about 1 inch (2.5cm) wide across your front hairline. Bring this section of hair up and past 90 degrees. You want it to stand straight up in line with your forehead. Insert the comb at the base of this section, and tease your hair, gently pushing the comb back through your hair about three or four times until it stands up on its own.

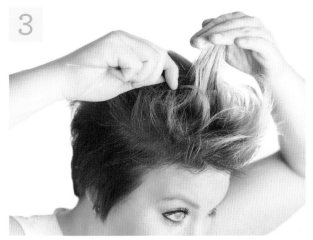

3 Move to another 1-inch (2.5cm) horizontal section of hair right behind the first one, moving backward away from your hairline. Repeat step 2.

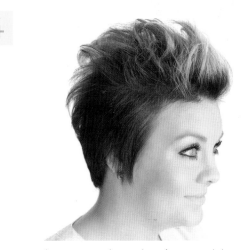

4 Continue with steps 2 and 3 until you've teased the entire top portion of your hair.

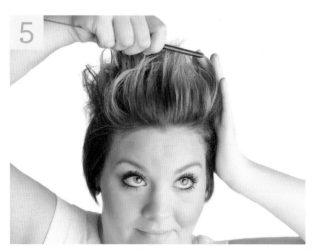

Use the rattail comb to gently comb back and mold your pompadour. You want a soft but edgy look. Be sure not to push to harshly into the areas you've just teased, however. You don't want to flatten down the hair you've just worked to volumize.

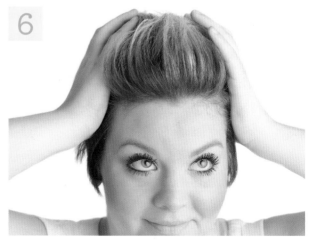

You can use a molding paste and/or a shine spray to further style your pompadour. Or you can mix them together to create a paste to tame unruly flyaways. Whichever you use, rub it into your palms and gently glaze over your pompadour to mold it into the shape you desire.

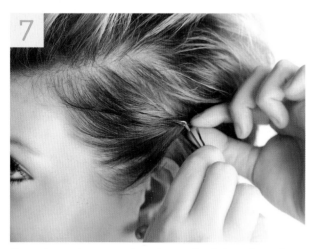

If your hair is longer on the sides, pin back the sides with bobby pins to enhance the height of your pompadour.

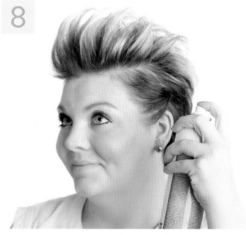

Set your hair with a medium- to firm-hold hairspray. You can use some additional shine spray to add a youthful glow to your coif.

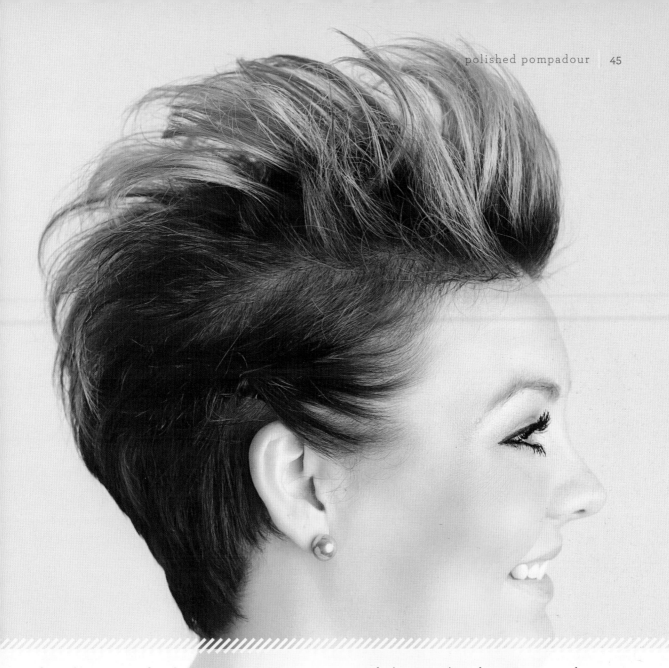

If you have extra-fine hair, you can use a $1^{1}/_{4}$- or 2-inch (3 to 5cm) curling iron to curl your top sections before teasing.

Longer-haired ladies can also achieve this look working with a U-shape section in the crown area. Use the rattail comb to section out your crown, starting and ending at your hairline's recession points. (Your recession points are located at the top corners of your front hairline, just above the outer corners of your eyebrows.) Then, comb your hair back into a medium to low ponytail bun, and create your pompadour as directed in the top section only.

Sleek Look

Short hair is commonly styled the same way day after day. Because of the length, oftentimes there's not a whole lot you can do with short tresses. So if you're looking to switch it up and add variety to your styling repertoire, this is the style for you. This sleek style works anywhere from a chic lunch with some girlfriends to the red carpet. You can wear this 'do styled wet or blown dry. The most flattering approach is to wear it with slight volume and blown dry. All hair types can sport this look; however, it's best suited for fine to medium hair types that are straight or wavy.

TOOLS NEEDED

blow-dryer

clips

concentrator

firm-hold styling gel

medium- to firm-hold hairspray

root lifter

round brush (You might need a variety of sizes for different results.)

water bottle

wide-tooth comb

PREPPING YOUR HAIR | Wash your hair with moisturizing shampoo and conditioner to help reduce frizz. If you have fine hair, be sure to thoroughly rinse the conditioner from your scalp. When drying, use a towel to get out the excess moisture, and gently wring your hair, not rub it. (Rubbing strands together can contribute to breakage.)

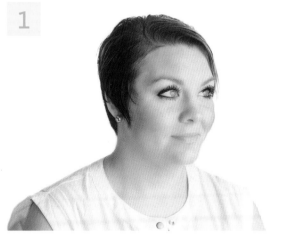

Start with towel-dried hair. Apply a root lifter to the hair at your crown area, spraying it directly at your scalp.

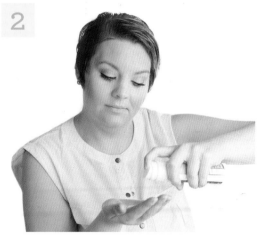

Next, apply a dollop of firm-hold styling gel about $^7/_8$ inch (2.25cm) to 1 inch (2.5cm) in diameter to the middle and ends of your hair.

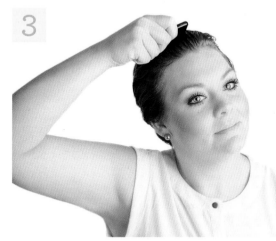

Use a wide-tooth comb to evenly distribute the product throughout your hair while gently detangling.

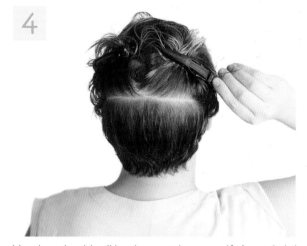

Your hair should still be damp at this point. If it's not, lightly spray it with a water bottle. Clip up all your hair except for a small horizontal 2-inch (5cm) section at the nape of your neck. If your hair is tapered at the neck, clip up all but the lowest 2-inch (5cm) layer you can clip.

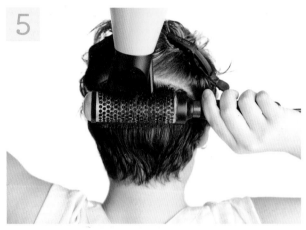

Insert a round brush underneath the bottom layer of the 2-inch (5cm) section, and hold your blow-dryer, with a concentrator attached, against the brush that's holding your hair. Blow-dry downward while rolling the ends for maximum body. Repeat, working around your head in the bottom layer, until your hair is dry. Unclip a second horizontal section, and repeat.

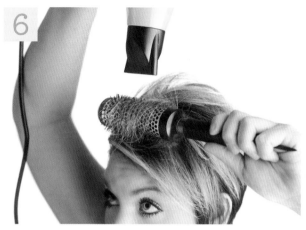

When you've reached the top section, insert the round brush at a 90-degree angle for maximum volume on top, and blow-dry.

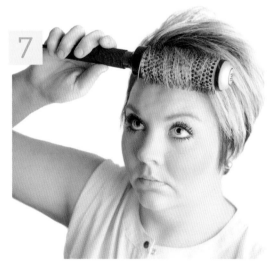

At your front hairline, working in a section 2 inches (5cm) wide, spray your hair with water if necessary to make it very damp. Hold the front section of hair outward at 90 degrees from your scalp. Insert the round brush underneath your hair, and blow your hair toward your face.

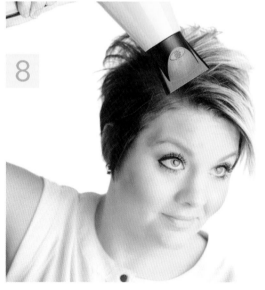

Repeat step 7 along the rest of your hairline on the sides, continuing to blow your hair toward your face while parting it on one side and pushing it slightly forward.

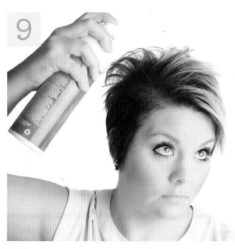

9

To finish, you can spray your hair with either a medium- or firm-hold hairspray. It's best to use an antihumectant hairspray for maximum hold so your style won't deflate.

If you like, you can tease the front of your hair and your crown for increased volume.

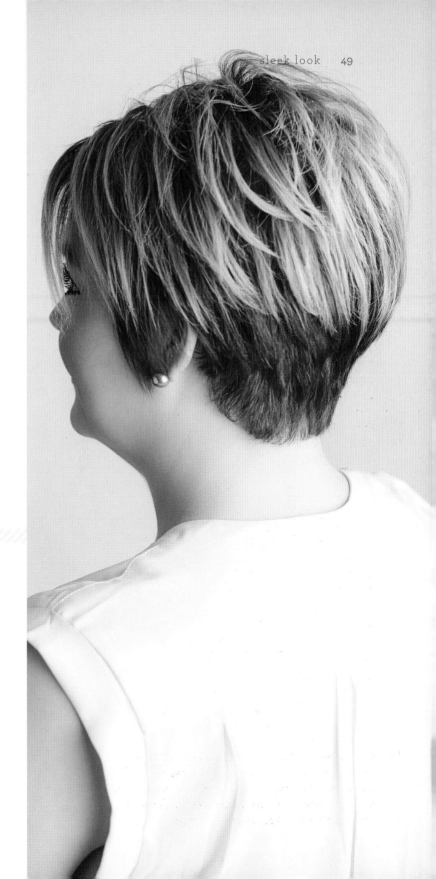

Curly Girl

This curly style enables you to have short hair that's versatile. It gives you the bounce and sass of short hair with the polish of a more sophisticated style. Picture wearing these soft coils more casually while out running daily errands or spiced up with a little volume for dinner and a movie. This style works with all hair textures. Naturally textured hair won't require as much prep time because this style can add curl and polish to what you already have.

TOOLS NEEDED

blow-dryer

clips

comb

concentrator

curling cream

curling iron with a 1-inch (2.5cm) barrel (or your preferred size)

defining paste

finishing spray

paddle brush

round brush (optional)

shine spray

PREPPING YOUR HAIR | If you have straight hair, use volumizers to plump up those strands and give your tendrils something to grasp on to. Wavy and curly textures can use a moisturizing serum when damp and a light-hold product, such as a sculpting or setting lotion or volumizing mousse afterward.

1

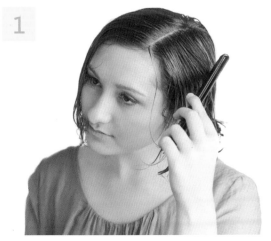

Start with thoroughly towel-dried hair that's slightly damp. Apply product as necessary, depending on your hair type, and gently comb through your hair with a comb or paddle brush. Prepping your hair before you blow-dry is vital to the finished style.

2

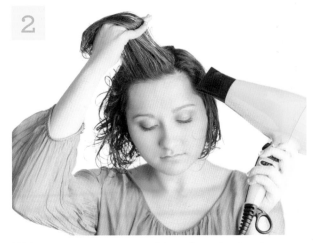

With a concentrator on your blow-dryer, dry your hair in opposite directions for volume. Remember to also continue drying your hair from the roots to the ends while you're flipping your hair back and forth. This helps smooth out knots and flyaway hairs.

3

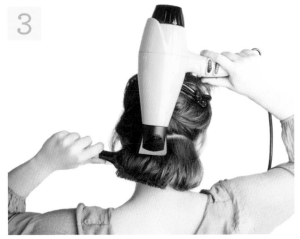

Most of the time when working with short hair, it's unlikely that you'll need to curl the area at the nape of your neck. It's best to try to smooth that area while you're blow-drying. You could add some slight shape there by inserting a round brush underneath your hair and rolling it down the back of your head.

4

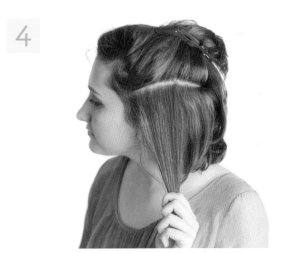

On whichever side your part is *not* on, divide that section in half. Clip up the hair on the top section of your head.

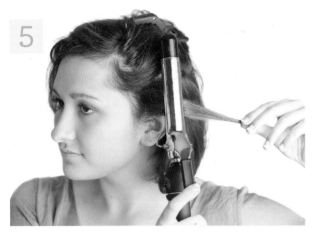

Insert a curling iron halfway down your hair, holding it open and at a 90-degree angle from your scalp. Be sure the curling iron clamp faces forward, so you're curling away from your face.

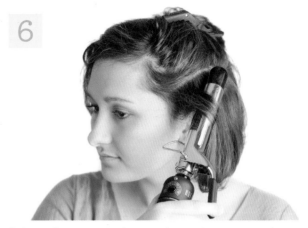

Release the spring so the iron clamps down on your hair in the middle. Roll the curling iron up your strand to curl the hair closest to your scalp and then gently glide it down your hair, toward the ends. Near the ends, loosen the tension on the curling iron just a bit so you're still holding the hair but you're moving closer to the ends, and roll it back up toward the roots. This enables you to curl your whole strand of hair in one step. Loosen the curling iron clamp, and release your hair until the iron is almost to the end of your hair. Then roll it up again.

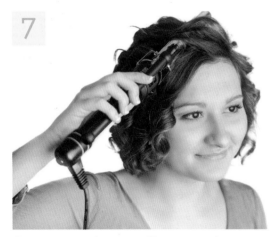

Grab another subsection of hair next to the one you just curled and repeat steps 5 and 6. After you've curled that subsection, release the section above and continue curling.

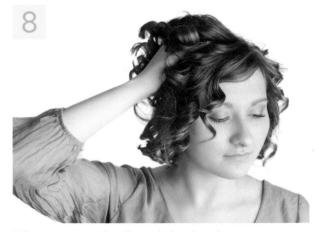

When your entire head is curled and cool, you can use a defining paste or curling cream to add polish to your curly locks. Squeeze a dollop about $3/4$ inch (2cm) to $7/8$ inch (2.25cm) in diameter into your palm, and rub your hands together until all you see is a slight sheen. Gently work the product through the middle and ends of your hair.

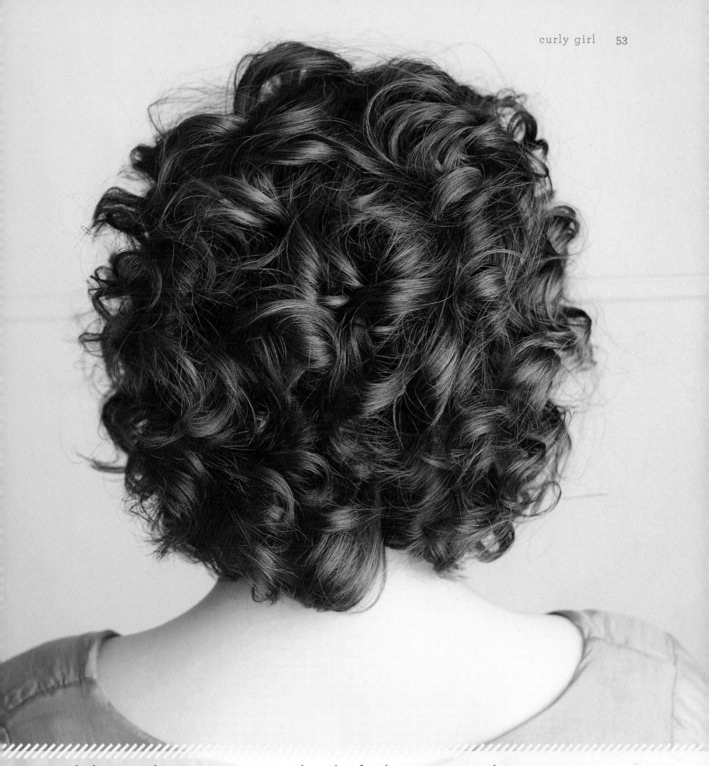

For a little more glamour, spray your curls with a finishing spray or a shine spray.

Side Swept

Side swept hair, or hair styled in a deep side part, has been shown frequently on longer-length hairstyles. But that monopoly is over! Carving your hair into a dramatic side part is a fresh and fun way to wear a shorter style. We're not talking comb-over status here, but deeper than an off-center part. If your hair is cut asymmetrically, the deep part can enhance the drama of your edgy mane. All textures and lengths can play with the side swept look. This version just happens to be specifically for the shorter end of the hair-length spectrum.

TOOLS NEEDED

blow-dryer

clips

concentrator

large boar bristle round brush

molding cream or paste

paddle brush

PREPPING YOUR HAIR | If you have
straight strands, you might want to use a wet look for a modern take on this style. Use a firm-hold gel to maintain the style. For a softer look, you can use a light-hold styling mousse to amp up your hair's natural texture. If you have curls, first use a moisturizing serum and then add hold with a gel or molding cream.

1

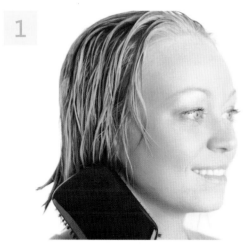

Start with thoroughly towel-dried hair. Apply product as necessary, depending on your hair type, and gently brush through your hair with a paddle brush.

2

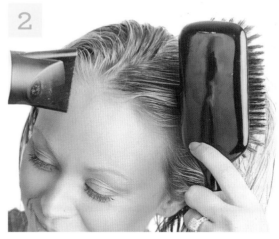

With a concentrator on your blow-dryer, use the paddle brush and dryer to blow-dry your hair from the roots to the ends in opposite directions to create soft volume.

3

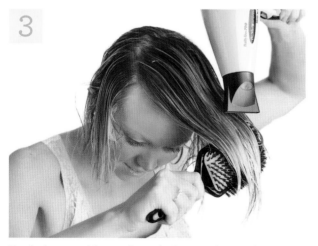

Brush down and forward on whichever side you choose to make your deep part. By continually moving your hair back and forth in a downward motion toward your face, you relax any cowlicks you might have in the front of your hair.

4

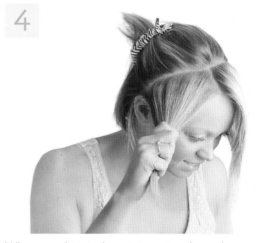

When your hair is about 80 percent dry, grab a small, horizontal section 1 to 1 $\frac{1}{2}$ inches (2.5 to 3.75cm) wide along your front hairline. Clip the rest of your hair back and out of the way.

Unless you're using a diffuser, it's always best to use a concentrator on your blow-dryer. The concentrator creates a stronger, more direct flow, which helps ensure a smoother style.

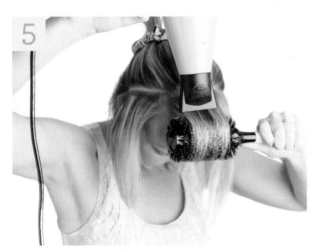

Using a large boar bristle round brush, smooth and tame your strands as you dry. Insert the brush underneath your front section of hair, and direct the heat downward with medium tension from the concentrator onto your brush. After you've gone down the section two or three times, move to the next section.

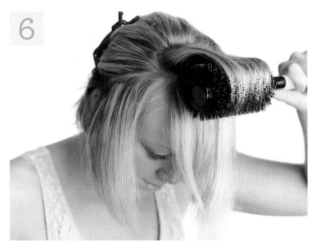

Grab a second horizontal section of hair behind the first, and repeat step 5 until your entire crown area is dry.

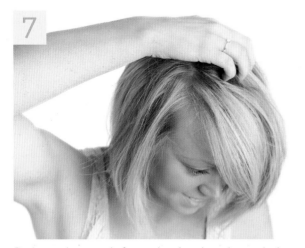

Push your hair gently forward and to the side on whichever side you prefer your part. Pulling your hair just slightly from back to front puts a contemporary edge to this classic style.

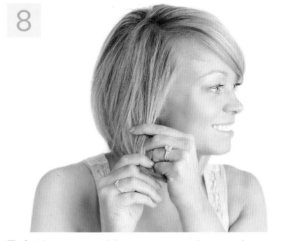

To finish, you can add texturizing products, such as a molding paste for fine hair to boost volume. If you have medium to thicker hair, add a softer molding cream to polish and tame your hair with a very light hold.

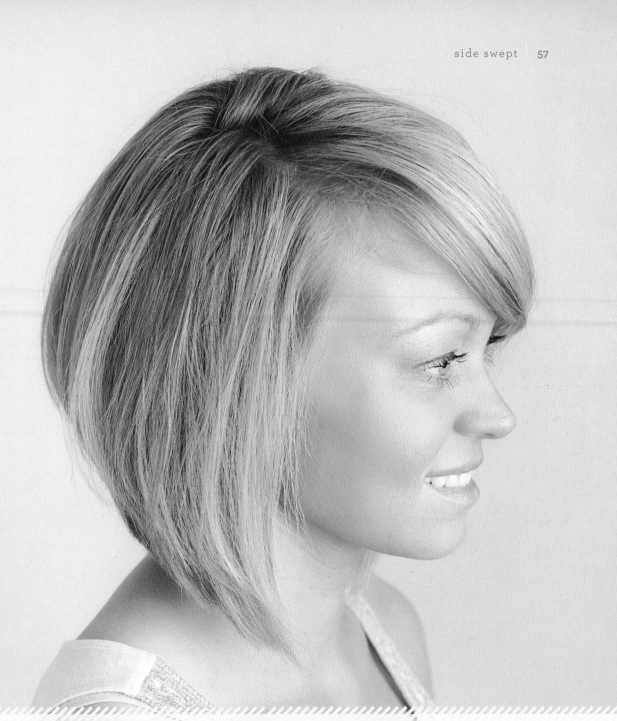

If you have curly hair and want to work with your natural texture, style as you usually would, but push your hair slightly forward and to the side when it's still damp. When your hair is dry, it's much harder to get any movement.

Short and Sassy Pony

The ponytail is a classic favorite. Whether you're going for a jog, volunteering at your favorite charity, or getting glammed up for a night out, the ponytail can transform to suit your needs. A shorter, spunkier version of the ponytail can fit your situation, too. The pony is easy, sure, but you don't want to look like you just rolled out of bed and threw your hair back. This style transforms the ordinary ponytail into something special—and a bit sassy!

TOOLS NEEDED

bobby pins

clear elastic band

clips

curling iron with a
1-inch (2.5cm) barrel

defining paste

teasing comb

working hairspray

PREPPING YOUR HAIR | If you have straight or wavy hair, prep your hair with a root-lifting spray for volume at the crown and a light-hold gel or mousse for the middle and ends of your hair. If you have curly hair, use a conditioning or moisturizing serum on the middle and ends of your hair, followed by a holding product such as a gel or mousse.

1

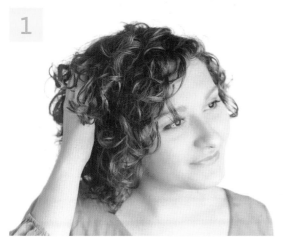

Start with dry hair that's been prepped with a light-hold product.

2

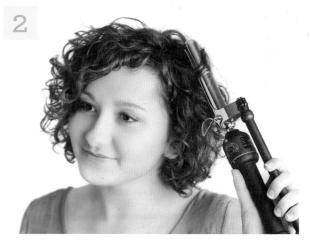

If your hair is shoulder length or shorter, use a curling iron with a 1-inch (2.5cm) barrel to add some texture.

3

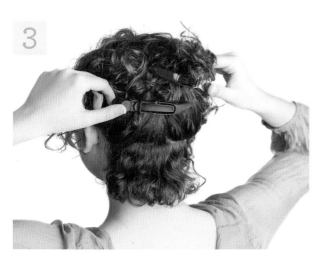

Part your hair where you normally part it. Leave about a 2-inch (5cm) section on the underside of your hair, and clip up the rest of your hair out of the way..

4

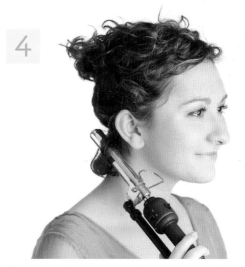

Use the curling iron to curl your hair away from your face. Your goal here is not to have perfect tendrils, but to add texture and movement to your hair. Be sure to curl all the way to the ends of your hair.

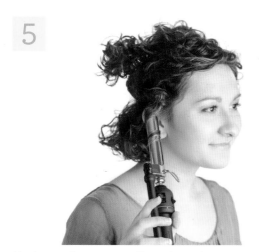

Unclip another section of hair above the section you just curled, and curl the new section away from your face. Repeat until your entire head is full of waves.

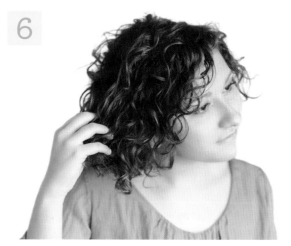

Gently rake through the waves with your fingers to soften them.

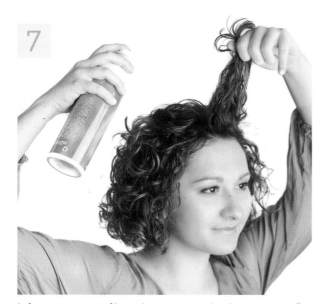

Lift up a portion of hair closest to your hairline in your bangs area, and spray it with a working hairspray.

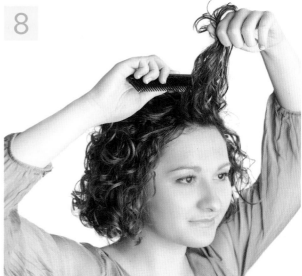

Gently use your teasing comb to create lift in the crown area. Repeat, working back toward the top of your head, to tease your entire crown.

9

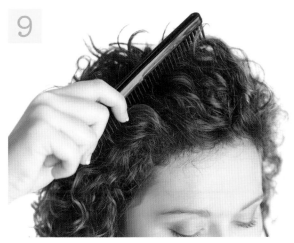

Use your comb to lightly comb over the area you just teased.

10

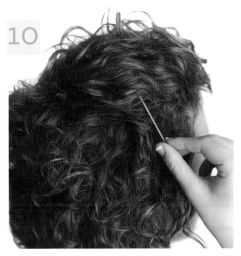

If your hair is short, use bobby pins to secure the loose ends that won't fit in your ponytail back and away from your face.

Is teasing bad for your hair? No, not if you do it correctly. The key is to use a teasing comb. This special comb enables you to create volume without damage.

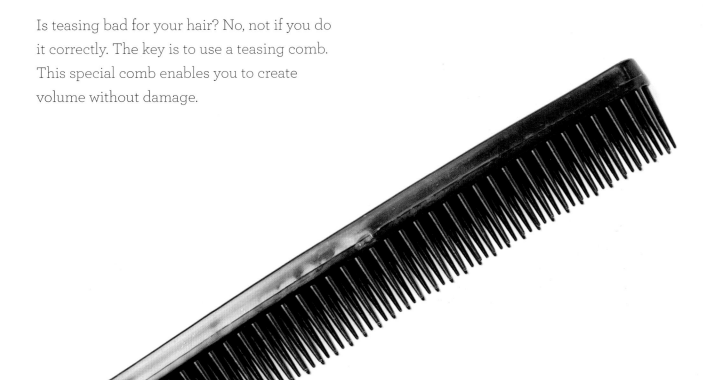

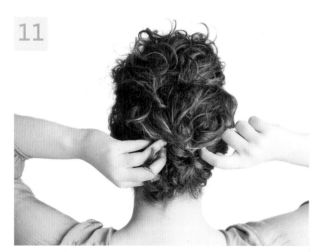

11

Gather your hair into a medium to low ponytail, and secure it with a clear elastic band. Your ponytail should look polished but not perfect. A little texture is necessary to add the sass.

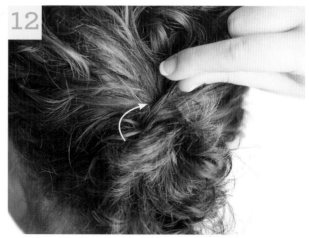

12

If your hair is long enough, wrap a small section of hair from your ponytail around the clear elastic band, and secure it with a hidden bobby pin under your ponytail.

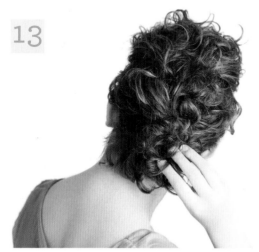

13

To add additional texture to the ends of your hair, squeeze a dollop of defining paste about $1/4$ inch (.5cm) in diameter into your palm. Rub your hands together and then scrunch the paste into your pony.

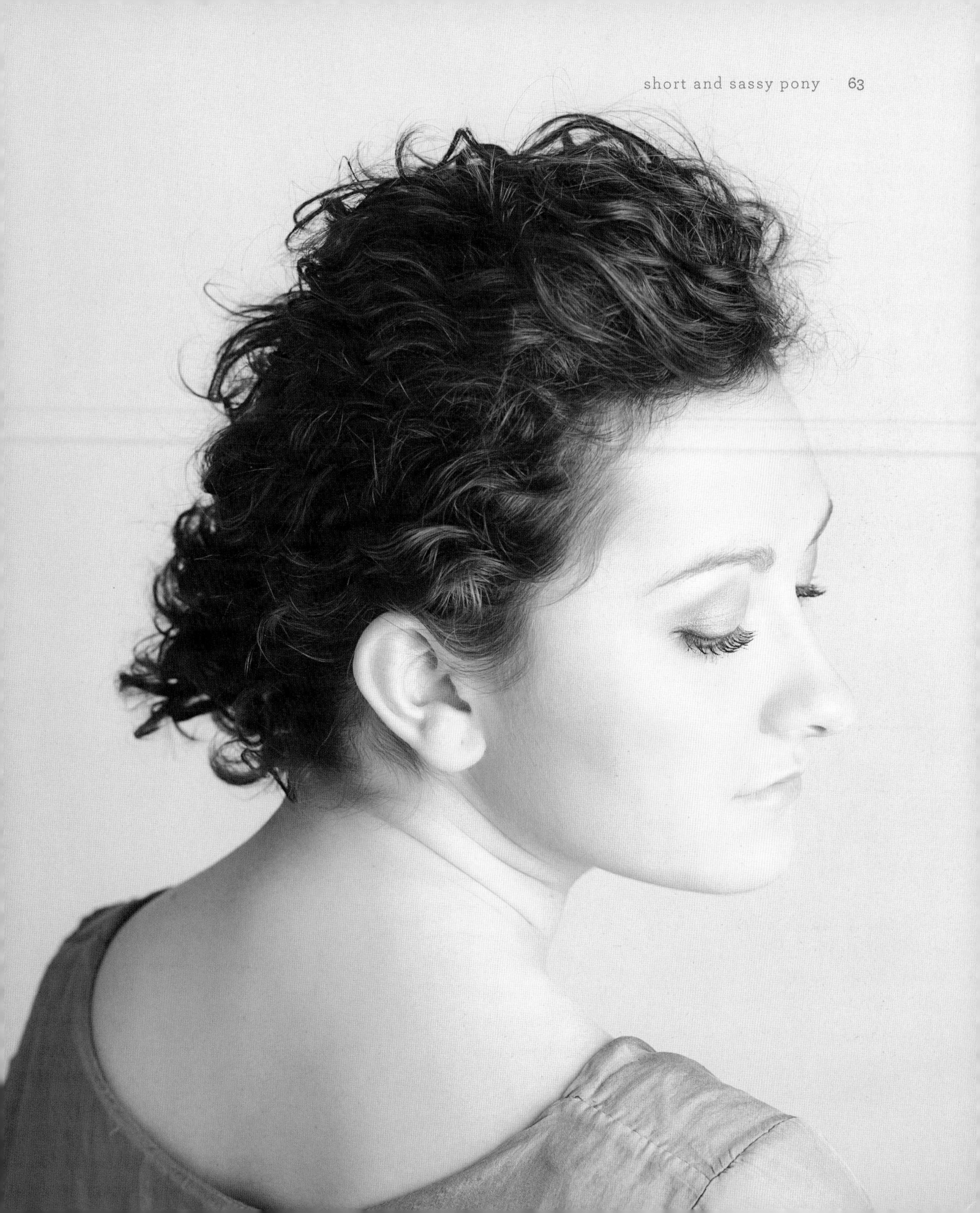

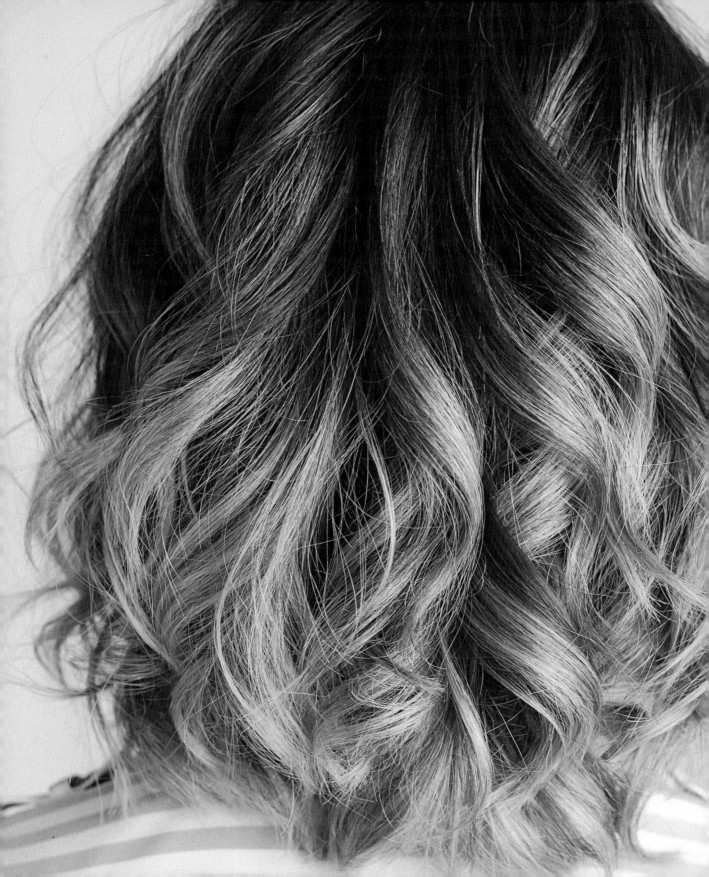

Styles for
MEDIUM-LENGTH
Hair

Medium-length hair is making a comeback, starting with the "Lob," or the "Long Bob," which you might have seen on the covers of your favorite magazine recently. Formerly, medium-length hair was all too often thought of as an in-between stage between a short cut and the longer length you really wanted your hair to be. And because it was a temporary look, it wasn't always styled in a current fashion.

There's good news for you medium-length ladies! Times have changed, and new, fresh medium hairstyles are easy to create, giving you lots of options to wear casually to the ballpark or dressed up for a night out on the town. These new and updated styles will have you loving your mid-length coif.

Basic Blowout

If you've ever wanted salon-worthy hair in the comfort of your own home, this easy style is for you. The Basic Blowout is meant to look polished yet effortless. It's a perfect style for every day but is also professional enough to be worn to the office or even to an after-work party. This versatile style works with many types of hair. You'll be ready to walk out the door in less than 30 minutes with the correct use of product and styling tools.

TOOLS NEEDED

blow-dryer
clips
concentrator
light-hold hairspray
paddle brush

round brush (The smaller the size, the more curl at the bottom.)
smoothing serum or paste (optional)

PREPPING YOUR HAIR | Your hair

should be thoroughly towel dried before you apply any product. If you have fine hair, use a cocktail of root lifter and volumizing mousse for some extra bounce. If you have medium to thicker strands, add volume and hold with a light-hold gel or styling glaze, and combat any frizz with a smoothing serum. If you have thick, coarse, or curly tresses, focus first on softening with a moisturizing serum and follow up with a mousse or gel for hold and shine.

1

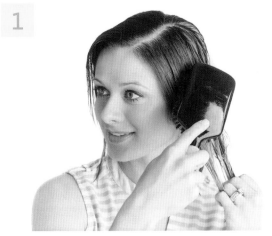

Start with thoroughly towel-dried hair. Apply product as necessary depending on your hair type, and gently brush through your hair with a paddle brush.

2

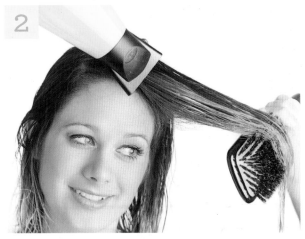

Fit a concentrator on your blow-dryer, and use the paddle brush and your dryer to blow-dry your hair from the roots to the ends in opposite directions to create volume until it's about 80 percent dry.

3

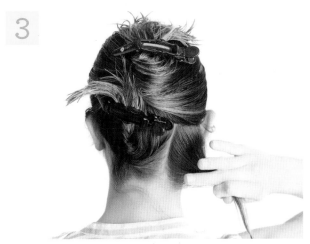

Clip up all your hair except for the bottom layer, and divide that bottom layer into 2-inch (5cm) horizontal subsections.

4

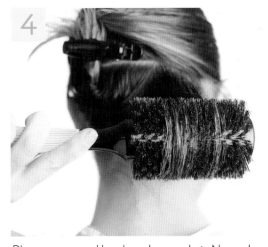

Place your round brush under your hair. Next, place your blow-dryer, with the concentrator, on top of the round brush, directing the heat downward. Turn your blow-dryer on medium heat, and direct the brush and concentrator down your hair in a steady motion with medium to high tension.

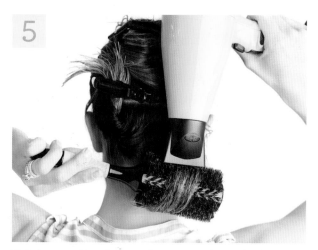

Roll the round brush a couple times on the ends of your hair with the heat still on it. Remove the blow-dryer, while the round brush is still rolled in your hair, and let it cool for 5 seconds before dropping the section.

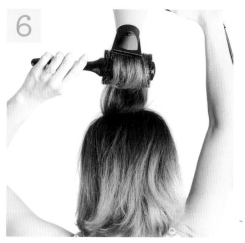

Repeat drying and rolling around your head. When you finish that section, drop another section from the next layer up, and repeat drying until you reach the top section at the crown of your head.

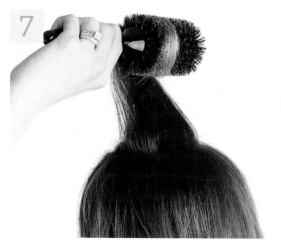

For added volume in your crown area, place the round brush under your hair and the blow-dryer on top, pulling with tension at a 90-degree angle from your scalp. Repeat steps 3, 4, and 5 until your hair is dry.

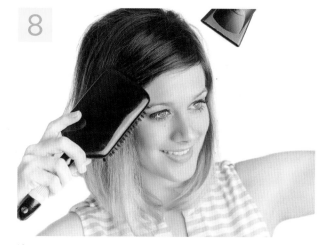

If you have bangs, dry them using a paddle brush while your hair is still damp, blow-drying in a downward motion. Moving your hair left to right, while still downward, helps reduce any cowlicks. Continue with steps 3, 4, and 5 until your fringe is fully dry.

9

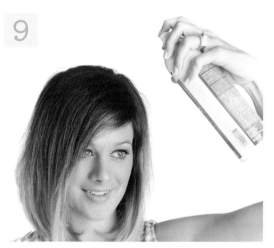

Set your hair with a light-hold hairspray. If you have textured or damaged hair, you might require a smoothing serum or paste to help tame frizz and flyaways.

If your hair tends to dry quickly, you can dry your bangs first, before step 1. Also, if you have stubborn cowlicks, this is also a good option to make them lay how you want them to.

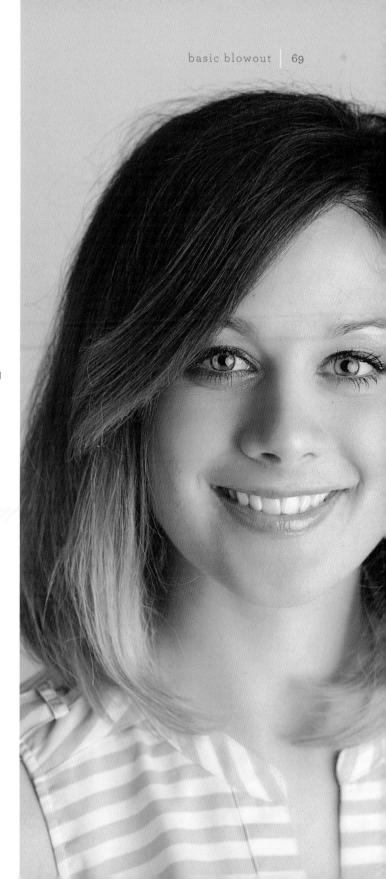

Flipped Out

This fun style lets you get creative with your hair, with the top portion turned under and the bottom section flipped up. Your turned-up hairstyle can be a fun new way for you to incorporate this fashion into your work day or out shopping with the girls. Most hair types will find this style easy to work with. If you are blessed with a little bit of natural bend, your tresses may stay "flipped" a bit longer.

TOOLS NEEDED

blow-dryer

clips

concentrator

light-hold defining paste

paddle brush

root booster

round brush (The smaller the size, the more curl at the bottom.)

sculpting lotion

volumizing mousse

PREPPING YOUR HAIR | It is best to

begin with a root-lifting spray and volumizing mousse for fine to medium hair types. For thick hair, use a combination of moisturizing serum and a light-hold gel or mousse afterward.

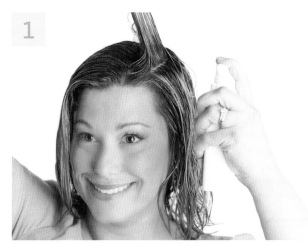

Start with thoroughly towel-dried hair. Add a volumizing mousse and/or sculpting lotion, with some root booster for extra flair.

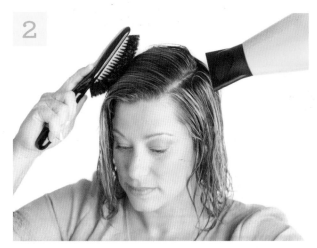

Using your blow-dryer with a concentrator attached, paddle brush your hair while moving in opposite directions to smooth and tame your tresses.

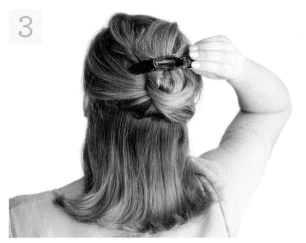

Divide your hair into two sections, one on top and one on bottom. Clip up the top section out of your way.

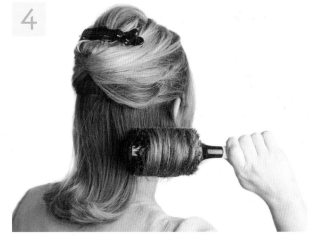

Push your round brush on the top of the bottom section of hair while rolling the brush upward.

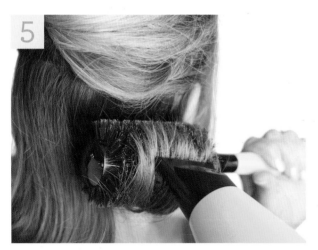

Spin the brush when you reach the ends, keeping the blow-dryer blowing from the roots to the ends.

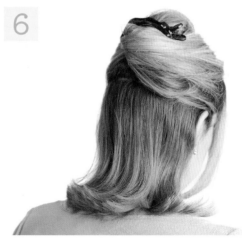

Repeat steps 4 and 5 until the bottom section of your hair is all flipping upward.

Never blow hot air *up* your hair shaft. This can cause major damage and frizz.

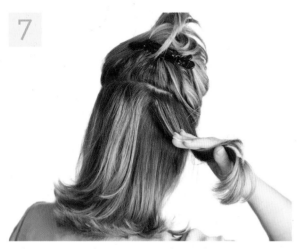

Release a horizontal subsection from of the top, clipped-up section of hair, and let it rest just above the flipped-out pieces underneath.

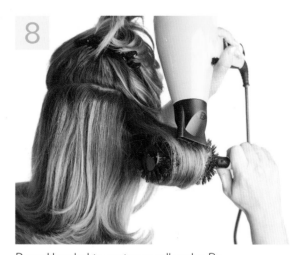

Round brush this section to roll under. Be sure to push with high tension while using the concentrator and the round brush, and roll a few times on the ends of your hair for extra bounce.

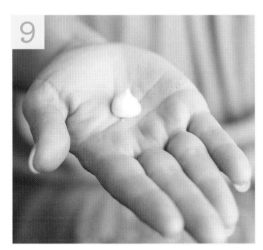

9

To finish, squeeze a dollop about $^3/_4$ inch (2cm) in diameter of light-hold defining paste into your palm. Rub the paste in your hands before applying it to your hair. This creates flow and separates your new sassy hairdo into body-boosting pieces for more volume and movement.

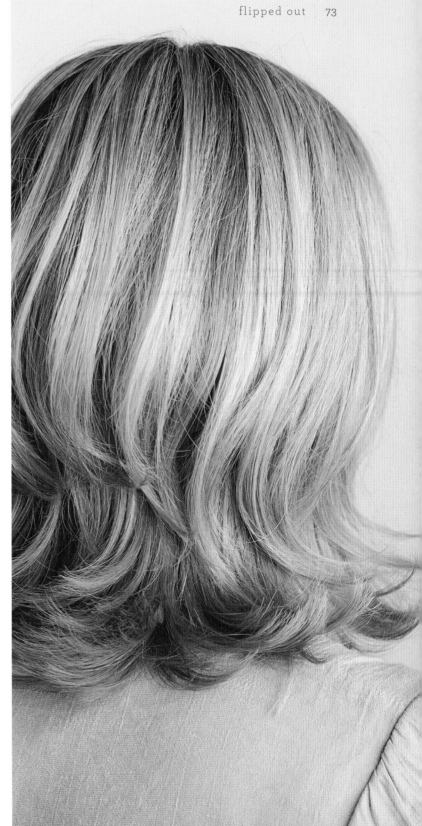

Beach Waves

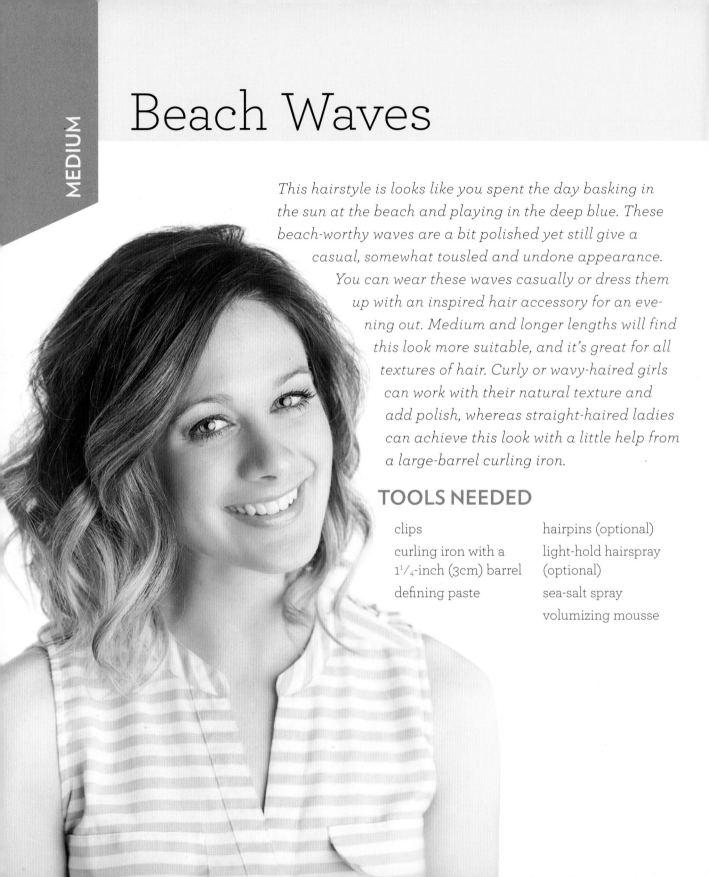

This hairstyle is looks like you spent the day basking in the sun at the beach and playing in the deep blue. These beach-worthy waves are a bit polished yet still give a casual, somewhat tousled and undone appearance. You can wear these waves casually or dress them up with an inspired hair accessory for an evening out. Medium and longer lengths will find this look more suitable, and it's great for all textures of hair. Curly or wavy-haired girls can work with their natural texture and add polish, whereas straight-haired ladies can achieve this look with a little help from a large-barrel curling iron.

TOOLS NEEDED

clips

curling iron with a 1¼-inch (3cm) barrel

defining paste

hairpins (optional)

light-hold hairspray (optional)

sea-salt spray

volumizing mousse

1

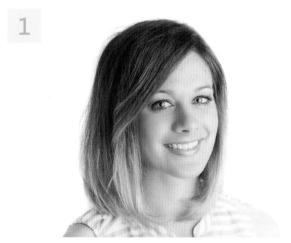

Start with towel-dried or dry hair. Add a texturizing product such as a sea-salt spray or volumizing mousse, and dry naturally for curly or wavy hair textures.

2

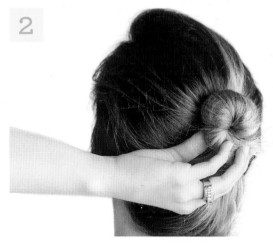

If you have straight hair, you can create a bit of texture by adding product, gathering your hair in a high messy bun, securing it with hairpins, and letting it dry.

3

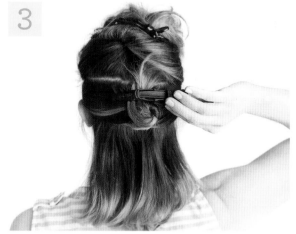

After your hair is completely dry and has some texture, separate it into three horizontal sections. Clip up the top two sections, and leave the bottom section down.

4

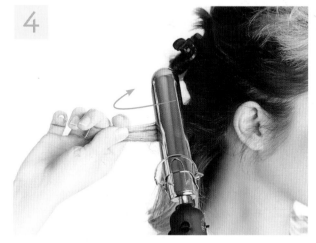

Hold a 1- or 2-inch (2.5- to 5cm) section of hair, starting closest to your face, at the ends with your fingers. Open the clamp of a $1^{1}/_{4}$-inch (3cm) curling iron forward, and place your hair between the barrel of the curling iron and the clamp, in the center of your strand. Close the clamp, and curl your hair away from your face.

5

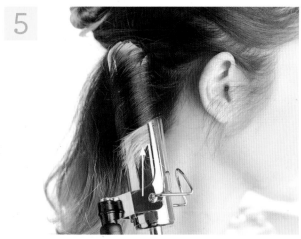

After you've curled that strand close to your scalp, push on the curling iron clamp to let a little hair slide out until about $^{1}/_{2}$ inch (1.25cm) of hair is left at the end of your piece of hair. Close the clamp, curl back up close to your scalp, and hold for 6 to 8 seconds.

6

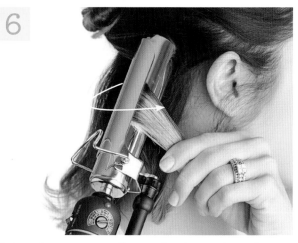

Pick up the next piece of hair, and curl toward your face using the same technique as steps 4 and 5 but now in the opposite direction. Repeat, curling in alternating directions, until all three sections of your hair are curled.

7

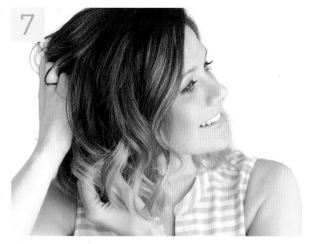

After your whole head has been curled, put a dollop about $^{7}/_{8}$ inch (2.25cm) in diameter of a texturizing product, such as a defining paste, in your palms, rub your hands together, and distribute it throughout your hair in a scrunching motion. This helps you comb out your curls, creating a beachy effect.

After you've combed through your hair with your fingers, you can spritz the sea-salt spray on your hair again for an extra tousled effect. For a more polished look, finish with a light-hold hairspray.

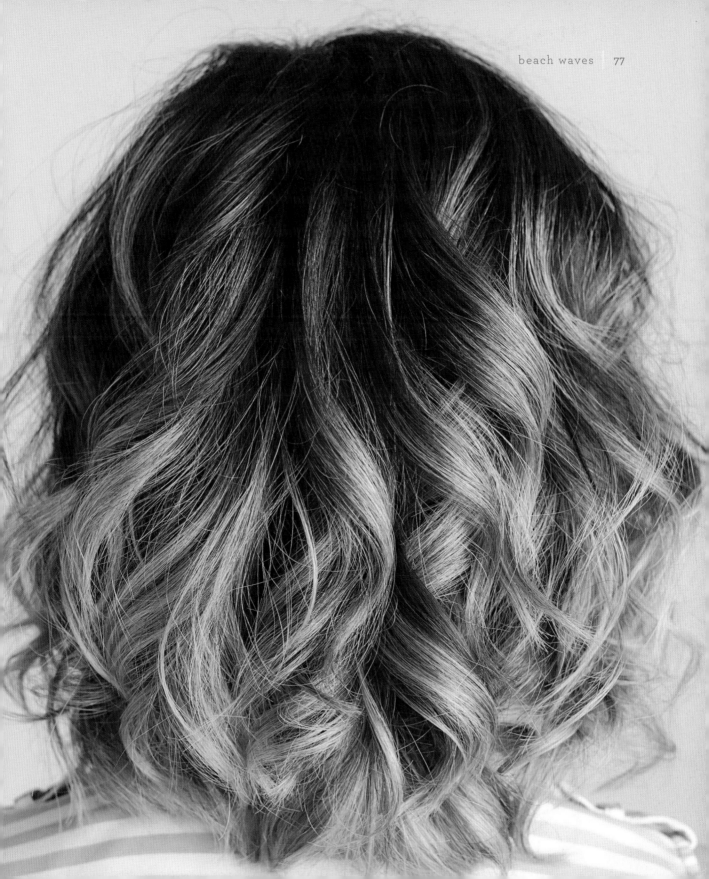

Polished Coils

Sometimes when you curl your hair, it doesn't always turn out like you expected. This style is a foolproof way to get polished curls that aren't too tight (think Shirley Temple style) or so loose they won't last past lunch. Polished Coils is great for everyday—wear it to work or when shopping with the girls—or even fancy enough for the annual charity ball. Medium- and long-haired gals will find this style most attainable.

TOOLS NEEDED

antifrizz serum (optional)

clips

curling iron with a 1-inch (2.5cm) barrel (or your preferred size)

defining paste (optional)

moveable-hold hairspray

shine spray

PREPPING YOUR HAIR | If you have
curly or wavy hair, use an antifrizz serum as well as a light-hold styling gel or mousse to retain the curl. If you have finer or straighter hair, you'll get the best results using a volumizer on your roots in your crown area for lift and a medium- to strong-hold gel or mousse on the ends of your hair to maintain the style.

1

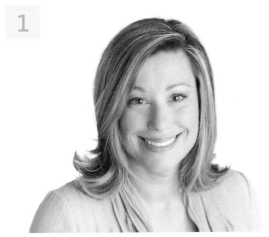

Start with hair that's been prepped with the proper products and blown-dry in opposite directions for volume.

2

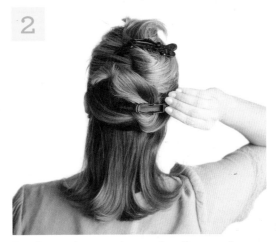

Divide your hair into three or four horizontal sections, depending on your hair's thickness. Leave the bottom section down for curling.

3

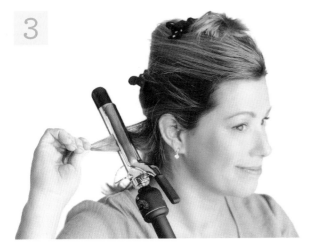

Start with a 1- or 2-inch (2.5 to 5cm) piece closest to your face, and hold it out perpendicular to your head. Open the clamp of a 1-inch (2.5cm) curling iron, facing forward, close it on your hair, and curl toward your scalp.

4

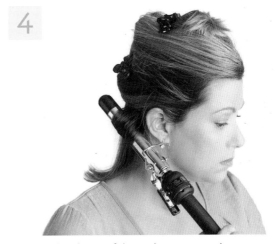

Push on the clamp of the curling iron to release some tension on your hair, and let the curling iron slide all the way to the bottom of your hair, Curl up one more time, all the way to your scalp, and hold for 6 to 8 seconds. Then drop the curl.

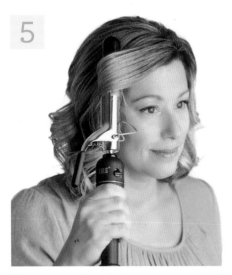

5

Continue curling the bottom section until you get to the center of your head. Starting on the opposite, front side of your hair, repeat step 4 again, curling away from your face. Continue curling until your entire head is curled. Let your hair cool for a few minutes.

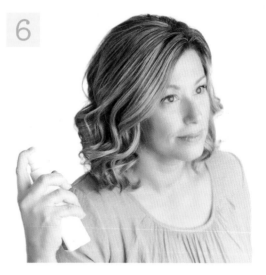

6

After your hair is cool, use a shine spray to mist your hair from your ears downward.

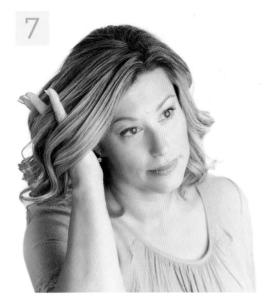

7

Rake your hands through your hair to loosen the curls.

If needed to tame frizz, you can use an antifrizz serum or a defining paste to add more polish to this style. For longevity, I recommend spraying with a moveable-hold hairspray.

The first time you try this style, it might take a little longer to divide your hair into the smaller sections and get your hands moving in the correct direction with the curling iron. Please don't get discouraged while you get the feel for this! When you master this style, you'll be able to complete it in a maximum of 10 minutes.

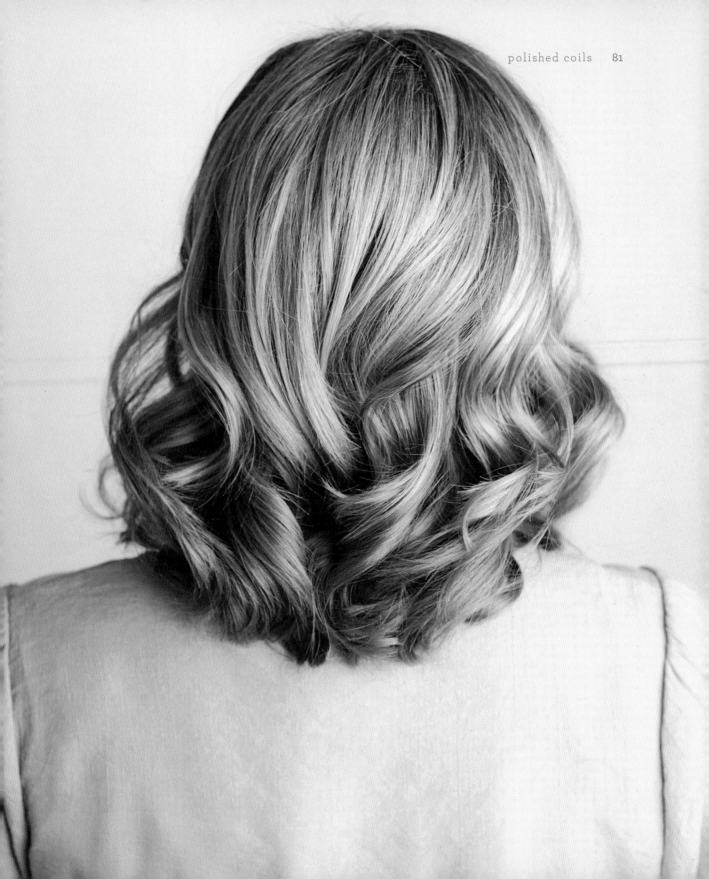

Undone Bun

All ladies with a little texture to their hair will adore this no-fuss style. If you aren't lucky enough to have any bend to your tresses, you can pump up the volume with a large-barrel curling iron. The undone bun is a quick, chic answer to bed head or a lazy Sunday afternoon. I picture this style out running errands or going to your kids' soccer games on the weekend. This bun can also easily transfer to evening with a deep side or center part and romantic pieces falling around your face.

TOOLS NEEDED

bobby pins

clear elastic band

curling iron with a 1$\frac{1}{4}$-inch (3cm) to 1$\frac{1}{2}$-inch (3.75cm) barrel

dry shampoo

teasing comb

PREPPING YOUR HAIR | If you're a
curly haired girl, prep your hair with an antifrizz product first and a hold product second. If you have wavy hair, you can intensify your texture with a sea-salt or waving spray and let your hair air-dry for extra oomph. If you have straighter strands, you can use root lifter and volumizing mousse for hold and fullness.

1

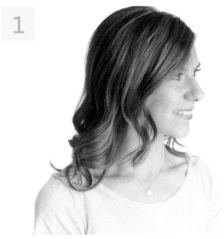

Start with dry hair, and use your large-barrel curling iron to curl your entire head of hair. (Sectioning is not important here. You're not looking for uniform curls, only texture.)

2

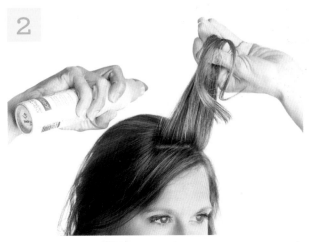

For a little extra volume on top, lift up your top, crown, section of hair, spray it with a dry shampoo for added texture, and tease with a teasing comb to create a little extra volume on top.

3

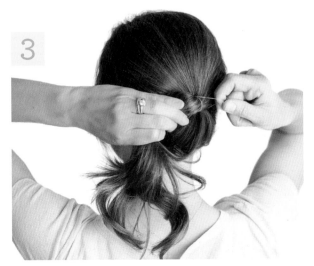

Gather your hair in a medium to low ponytail, and secure it with a clear elastic band. For extra volume, you can tease your ponytail at this point, too.

4

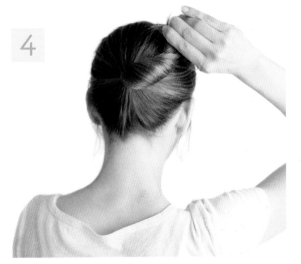

Twist your ponytail until it starts to bend. It will continue to bend around in a circular bun shape as you continue to twist.

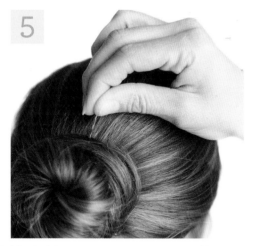

Use bobby pins to secure your twisted bun.

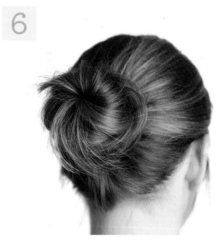

Pull out a few pieces of hair from the bun, and tuck them in and around your loop for added messiness.

You can use whatever size curling iron you like to add texture to your hair in step 1. If your hair is more of a medium length, use a curling iron with a $1^{1}/_{4}$-inch (3cm) barrel. If you have longer hair, you can use a curling iron with a $1^{1}/_{2}$-inch (3.75cm) barrel. And remember, your goal isn't picture-perfect curls but rather volumizing texture.

Give your finished style a retro vibe by adding a scarf or bandana around your head to showcase your bun. Or pull your ponytail and, therefore, your bun to the side.

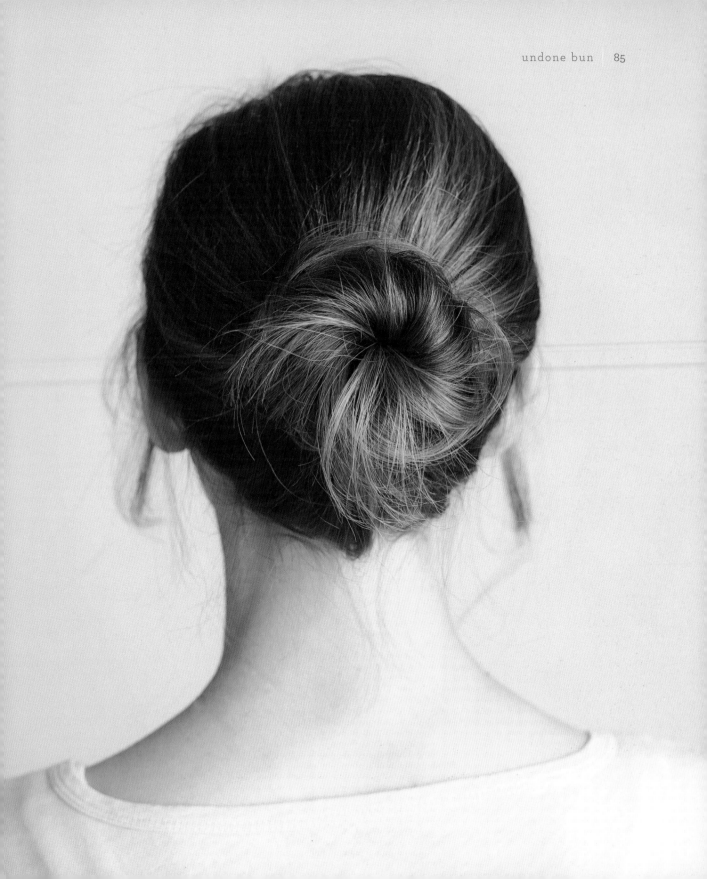

Party Pony

This isn't your average ponytail! The Party Pony is a volumized version of the original. This quick and easy style is great for a girls' night out, summer concerts, or a coworker's birthday party. All types of hair can rock this look; however, wavy and straight hair types will find this pony easier to do.

TOOLS NEEDED

bobby pin

clear elastic band

light-hold hairspray
or dry shampoo

teasing comb

PREPPING YOUR HAIR | When your
hair is dry, you can add a little extra movement with a
waving or curl-enhancing spray. If you have fine hair, use a
dry shampoo to get the necessary volume on the top.

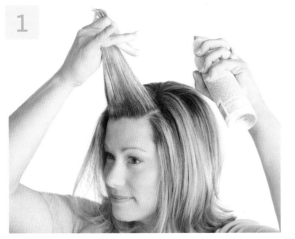

1

If you have bangs, lift them upward and spritz a light-hold hairspray or dry shampoo on the roots for grip.

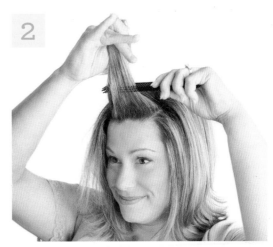

2

Starting with about a 3- or 4-inch-wide (7.5- to 10cm wide) and 1-inch-deep (2.5cm deep) section of hair near your hairline, lift a section of hair upward and tease with a teasing comb in a downward motion three or four times. Continue teasing small sections, moving back across your head, until you reach the top of your head.

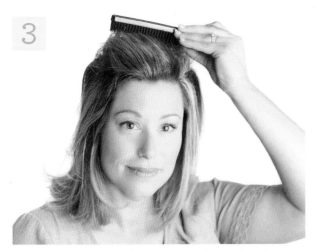

3

Comb over your teased area to smooth it and push your hair back away from your face.

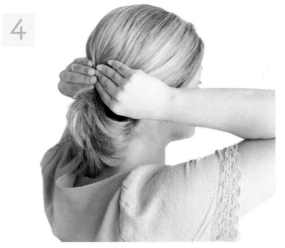

4

Gather your hair in a high or a low ponytail, being gentle with the top section so it retains plenty of volume. Secure your ponytail with a clear elastic band.

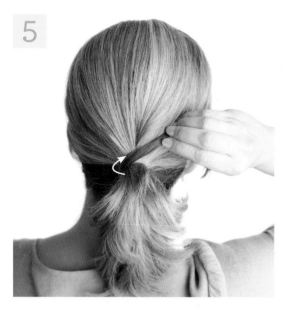

To cover the elastic band, take a piece of hair from your ponytail and wrap it around the elastic. Use a bobby pin to secure this piece of hair under your ponytail.

You also could use a rattail comb to create volume and added texture. Insert the comb in your teased crown, and pull upward with the end of the comb.

If you have curly or wavy hair and would like to try this style with straight hair, you can flat iron your hair before step 1 so you'll have a sleek and straight pony.

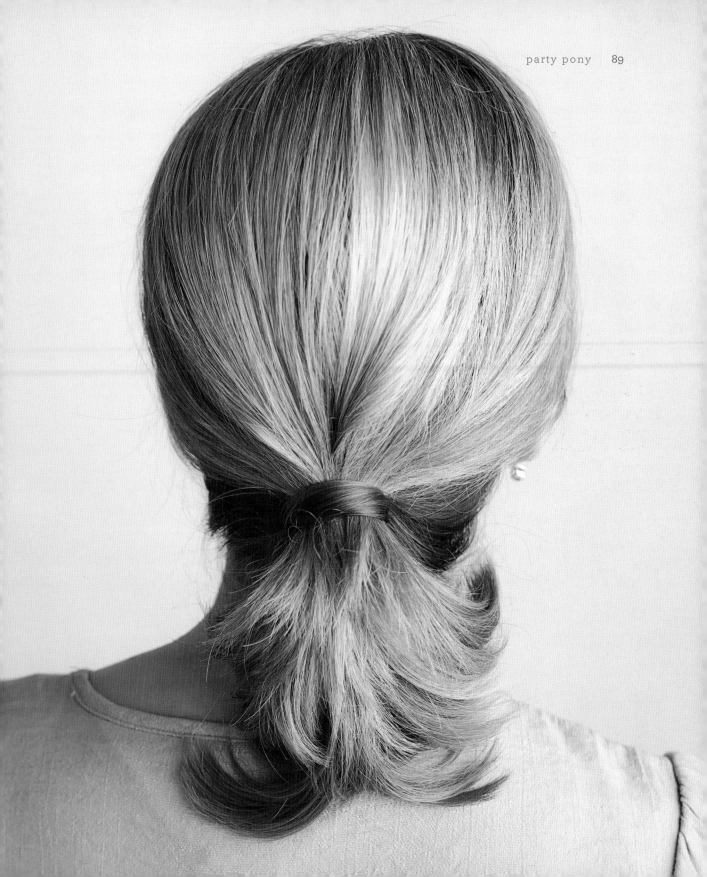

Braided Headband

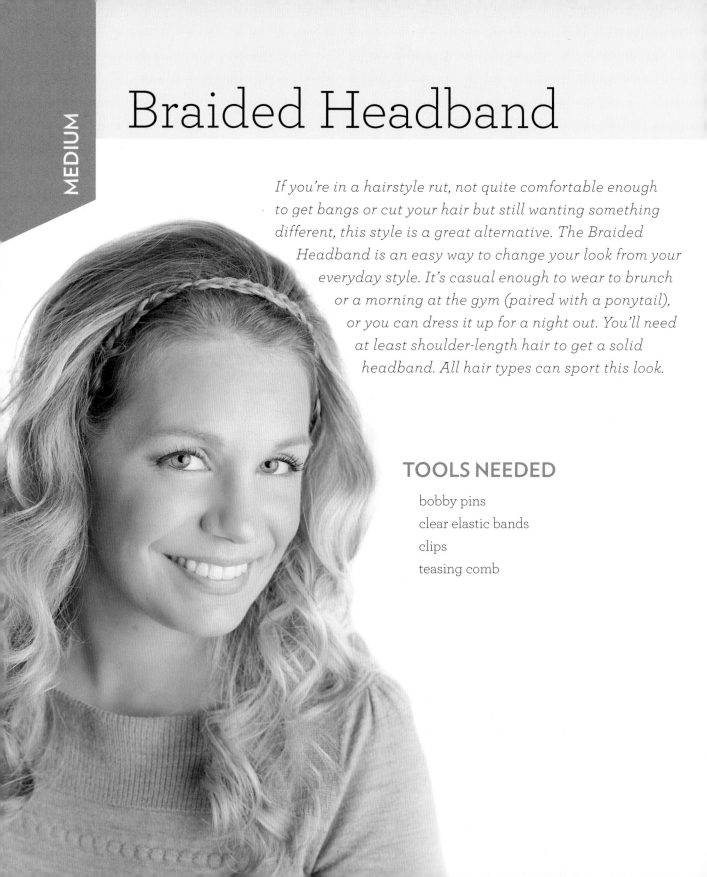

If you're in a hairstyle rut, not quite comfortable enough to get bangs or cut your hair but still wanting something different, this style is a great alternative. The Braided Headband is an easy way to change your look from your everyday style. It's casual enough to wear to brunch or a morning at the gym (paired with a ponytail), or you can dress it up for a night out. You'll need at least shoulder-length hair to get a solid headband. All hair types can sport this look.

TOOLS NEEDED

bobby pins

clear elastic bands

clips

teasing comb

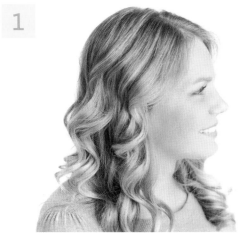

Start with dry hair in the style you prefer—curly, wavy, or straight.

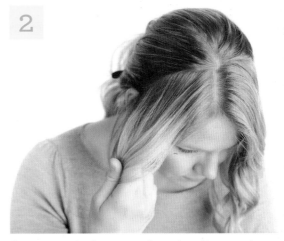

Section out the front part of your hair. Part your hair across your head from the top of one ear to the other, and clip the rest of your hair out of the way.

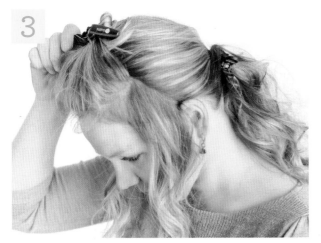

Part your hair again, this time separating the front section of hair left down. This section should span from the arch of your left eyebrow to the arch of your right. Tie back this section with a clip or clear elastic band. You should have two sections of hair hanging down now.

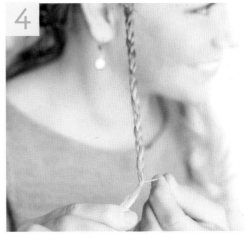

Working in the section of hair on the right, braid it to the bottom and secure the braid with a clear elastic band at the end.

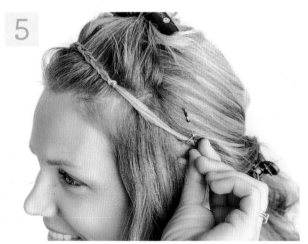

5 Wrap the braid you have just completed up and across your front hairline, leaving about a 1-inch (2.5cm) gap from your hairline. Secure this braid with bobby pins to hold it in place.

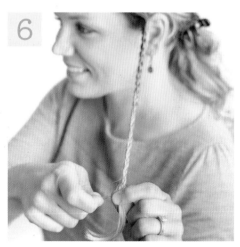

6 Braid the left section of hair as you did for the right side, and wrap the second braid up and across your head, right behind the first, creating a double braided headband.

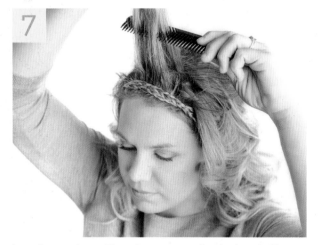

7 Let all your clipped hair down except for the braids. For extra volume and fullness, you can use a teasing comb to tease the crown section right behind your braided headband.

Instead of using braids, you could twist the lower sections of hair and wrap the twists around your head. Pin as directed to secure.

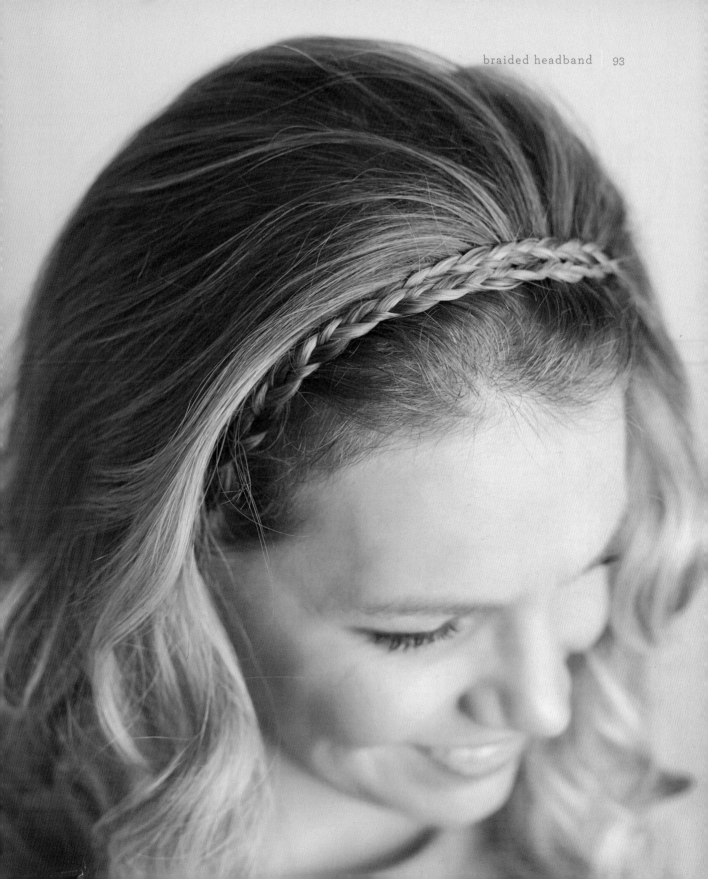

Inside-Out Pony

The ponytail has been around for ages and is due for an upgrade. Consider the Inside-Out Pony the average ponytail's more sophisticated older sister. Instead of a style you can quickly throw back to go run errands or get you through a serious sweat session at the gym, this pony can evolve to daytime wear. This 'do is elegant enough to wear to a business meeting, yet fun enough for a play date at the park. All hair types can wear this pony.

TOOLS NEEDED

antihumectant
hairspray
clear elastic bands

PREPPING YOUR HAIR | You can start this style with just about any texture in your hair—straight, wavy, or curly.

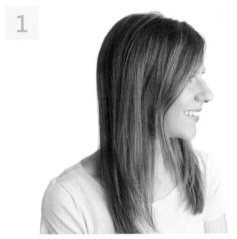

Start with dry hair.

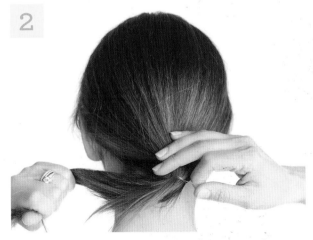

Gather your hair in a low ponytail, and secure it with a clear elastic band.

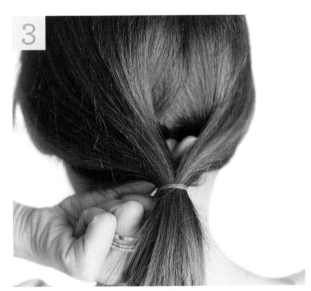

Reach up under your ponytail, and using two fingers, and make a hole in your ponytail, between your scalp and the elastic band.

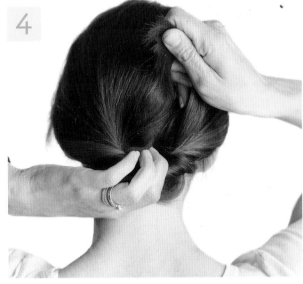

Reach through the hole from below, grab the base of your ponytail, and begin to pull your ponytail through the hole.

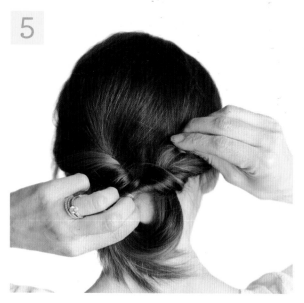

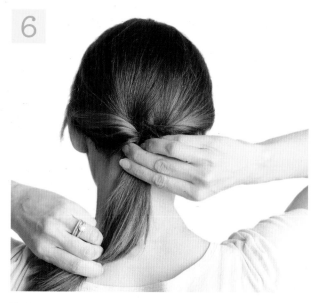

Continue to pull your ponytail through the hole to make it look inside out.

Tighten your tail by moving the elastic upward.

To set your hair, spray with an antihumectant hairspray for hold. Use a comb to carefully tame any loose hairs after you've sprayed.

To make your Inside-Out Pony a bit fancier, you can either braid your low pony or fishtail braid it before you turn it inside out. If you choose to use one of these adaptations, carefully cut the clear elastic band with scissors and remove it after the style is complete.

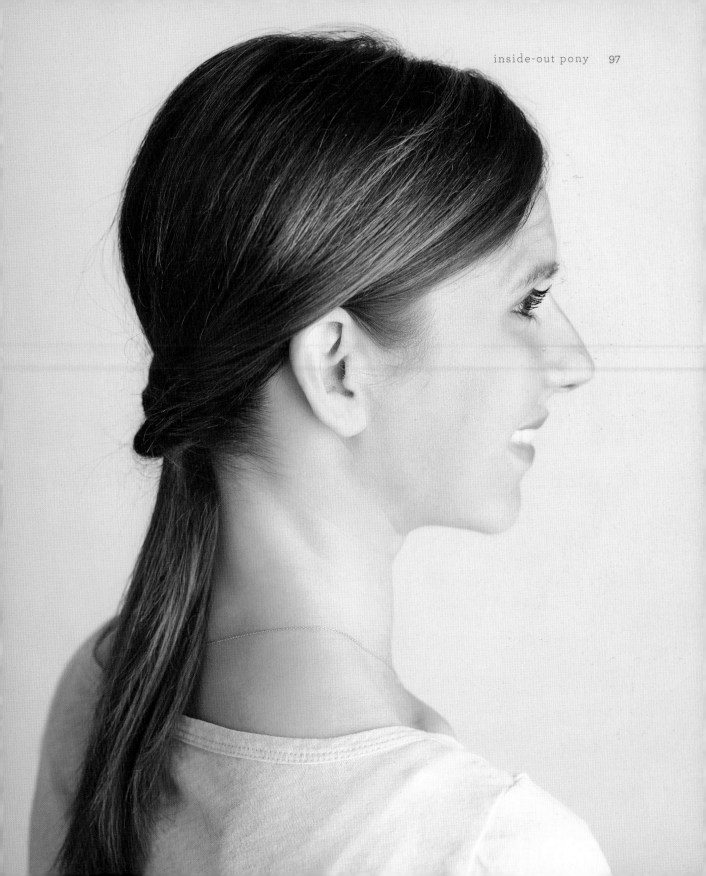

Upside-Down Braided Knot

If your ballerina bun needs an update, this style is for you. It's a funky, fresh adaptation of the top knot or braided bun you can wear just about anywhere. The Upside-Down Braided Knot can take you from the farmers' market to dinner with friends. For an extra touch of fun, you could add a hair accessory underneath the knot. All hair types can wear this style.

TOOLS NEEDED

clear elastic bands

clips

hairpins

medium- to firm-hold hairspray

PREPPING YOUR HAIR | You want some texture in your hair before you start this style. Slightly curly or wavy hair is best. If you have extremely curly locks, soften and smooth your hair a bit before beginning.

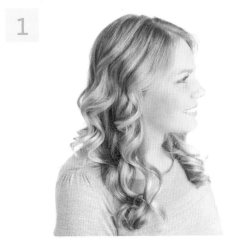

1

Start with dry hair.

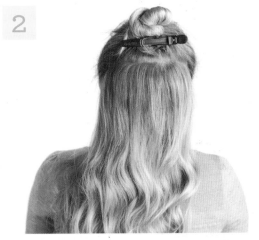

2

Divide your hair into two sections, parting it from ear to ear. Clip up the top section to keep it out of the way.

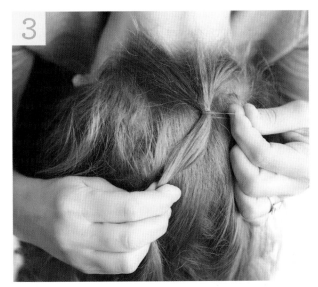

3

Tilt your head gently in an upside-down position. Grab a small section of hair at the nape of your neck to begin the French braid. If it's easier to manage, you can secure this small section with a clear elastic band for more control.

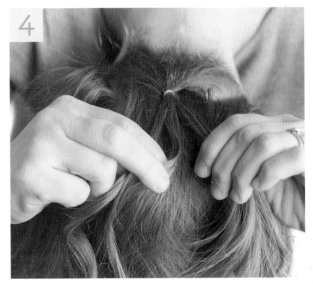

4

Divide the small section into three subsections.

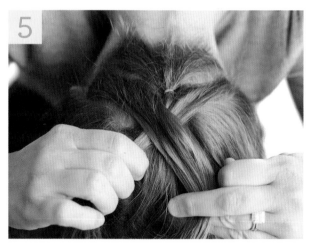

Fold the right side of the subsection over the center, still keeping the three sections separate. Then, fold the left side over the center, still keeping the three sections separate.

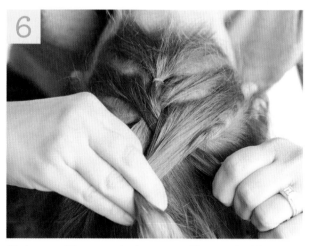

Grab a small horizontal subsection of hair, and add it to the piece that's now on the right side. Fold that section over the center.

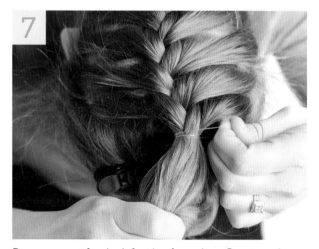

Repeat step 6 for the left side of your hair. Continue this process until you reach the top of your bottom section of hair. Secure the upside-down French braid with a clear elastic band.

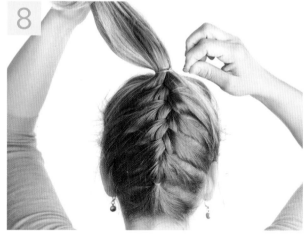

Tilt your head back to upright, and comb the top section of your hair back to meet the French braid. Combine the two sections into a high ponytail, and secure with another clear elastic band.

Before securing your hair in step 6, you can tease your crown area using a teasing comb. This is especially helpful if you have thinner hair.

9

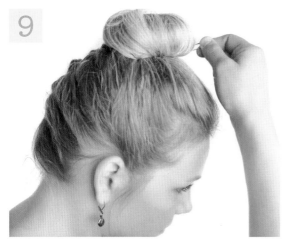

Lift upward on the ponytail, and give a slight twist. Wrap the pony around the clear elastic band into a soft bun, and secure with hairpins.

10

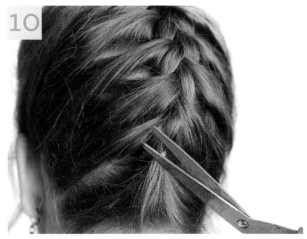

Cut and remove the first clear elastic at the base of your neck.

11

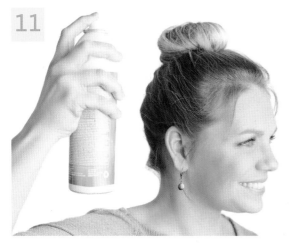

Finish with a medium- to firm-hold hairspray to secure your style.

To secure your bun with hairpins in step 9, insert a large hairpin into the bun, push it down into your hair, into the hair beneath your bun, and weave it back up into the bun. After you've weaved up and down a few times, gently push the hairpin into your hair.

Between steps 8 and 9, you can vary from the original bun instructions and braid your ponytail before wrapping it around the clear elastic band.

Finally, for an extra bit of fancy, wrap a ribbon around the base of the bun and tie it into a bow at the back.

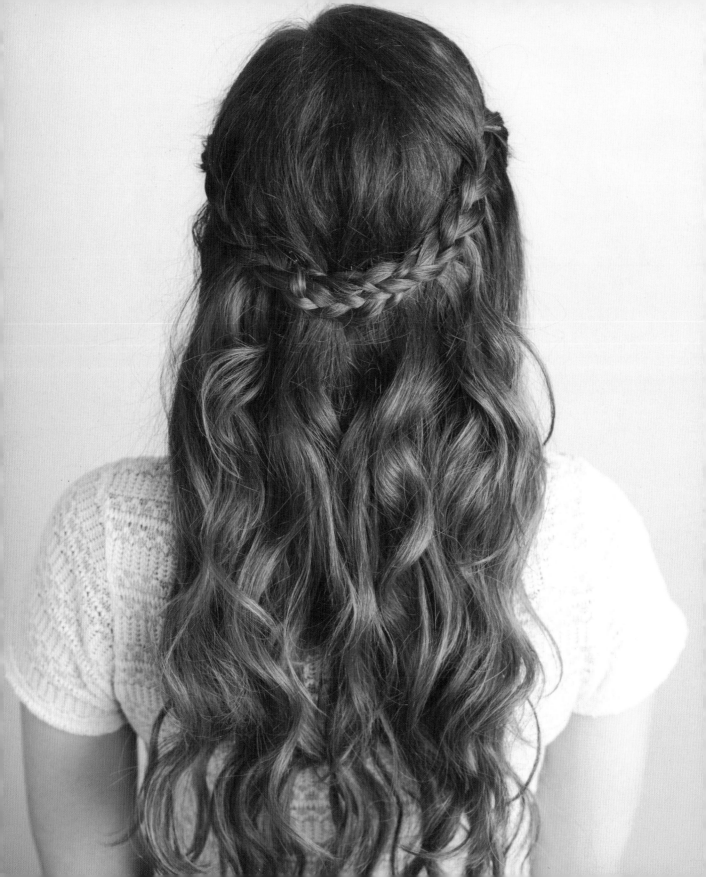

Styles for LONG Hair

Long hair is often the most versatile length of hair and can be braided, straightened, curled, teased, and twisted into a diverse number of styles. Starting with a technique as easy as a basic wave and leading to more intricate and eye-catching styles, the step-by-step directions for longer-length styles in this section will have you mastering your long locks in no time.

Throughout these styles, I share lots of tips and tricks to help you develop your hairstyling know-how. You'll enjoy trying new things with your hair—and keep it healthy and happy—if you first master the simple steps necessary to bring your hairstyle to life. And once you've mastered a few of the basics, I give you some more advanced styles to try when you're feeling ambitious!

Long hair isn't hard to style; it's simply a matter of taking the time to work through each style properly.

Basic Braid

The braid is a great hairstyle to learn because it can lead you to so many other styles. For a stylish but casual look, you can wear a braid low and on one side. Or you can use a braid to camouflage bangs you're trying to grow out. The braid offers countless variations when it comes to simple but sensational styles, and the Basic Braid is versatile enough to wear anytime or anyplace. It's suitable for all hair types.

TOOLS NEEDED

clear elastic bands
light-hold hairspray

PREPPING YOUR HAIR | While you're first learning how to braid, it's best to start this style with dry hair. When you get more comfortable with the technique, you can start it when your hair is damp or wet.

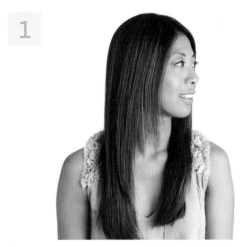

Start with straight, wavy, or curly hair.

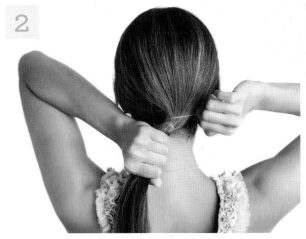

Gather your hair into a low ponytail, and secure it with a clear elastic band.

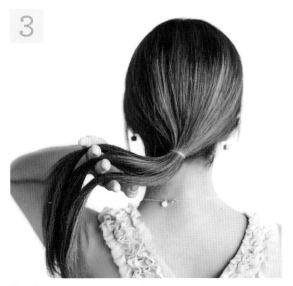

Divide your ponytail into three equal sections.

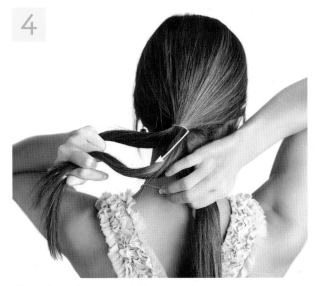

Cross the right section of hair over the center section, continuing to retain the three individual sections.

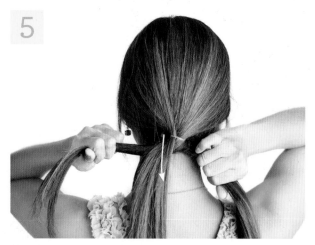

Cross the left section over the center section. (This is the section that was previously on the right side but is now in the center.)

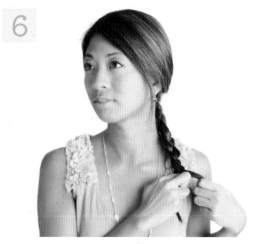

Continue steps 4 and 5 until you reach the end of your hair, and secure with a clear elastic band.

As you get farther down your braid, you can swing your hair over one of your shoulders so you can see it in the mirror as you work.

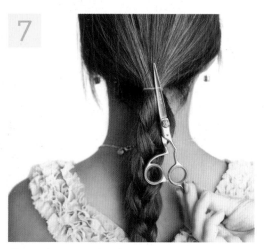

Cut and remove the elastic band at the base of your ponytail if you like.

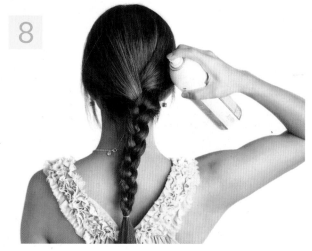

Finish with a light-hold hairspray.

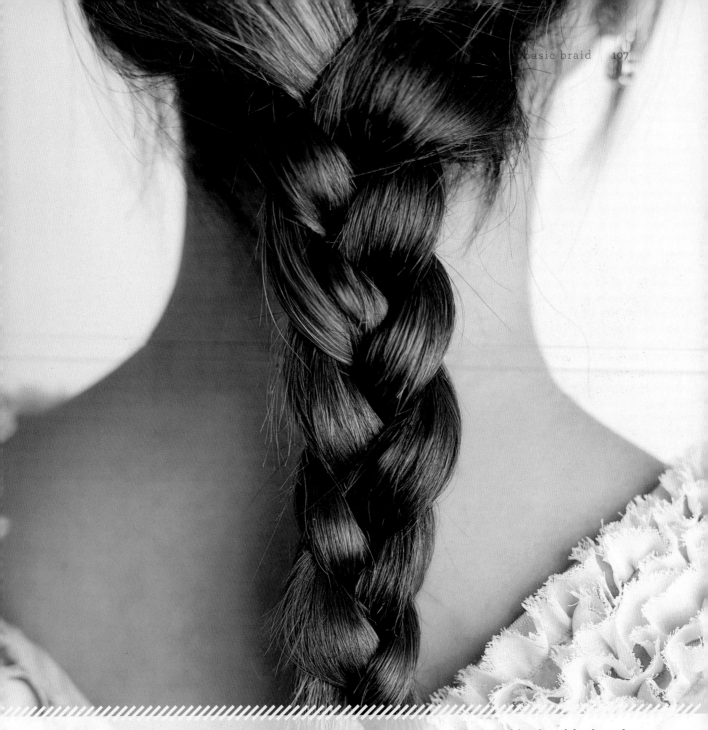

For quick and easy date night hair, tease your crown area for a disheveled look, add a braid, and voilà! You have sassy hair in no time. You also could curl your hair before braiding to give it a little extra texture if your locks are in need of more body.

French Braid

The French Braid is one of those hairstyles that looks harder than it really is. Once you've mastered this style, you can create many other versions stemming from the original design. This style is so easy to dress up or down; you can wear it for everything from a casual movie night at a friend's house to a prom or special event. Straight, wavy, and curly hair all work well with this braid.

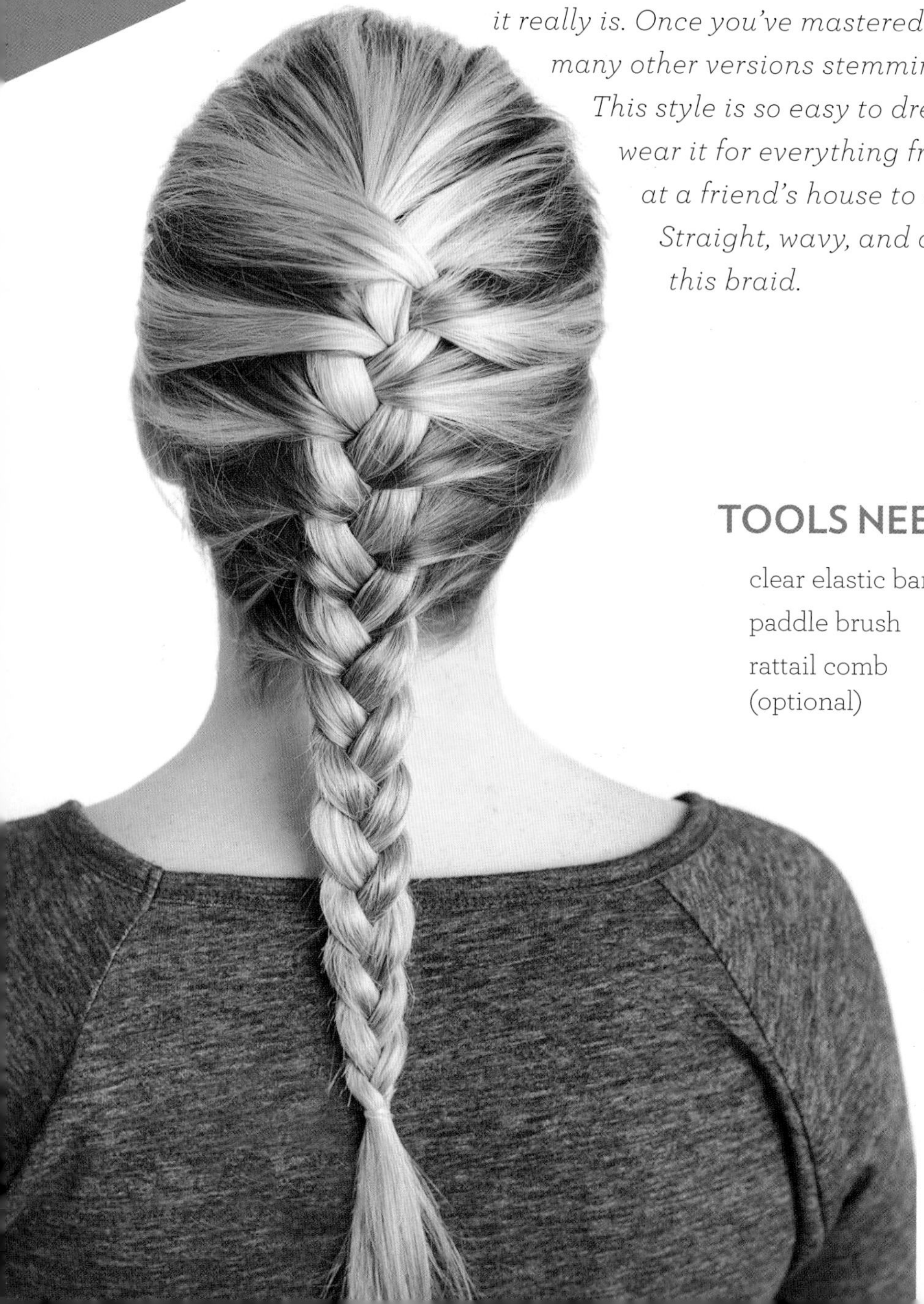

TOOLS NEEDED

clear elastic bands
paddle brush
rattail comb
(optional)

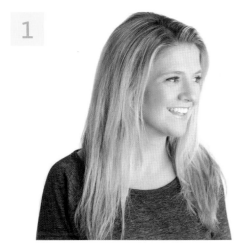

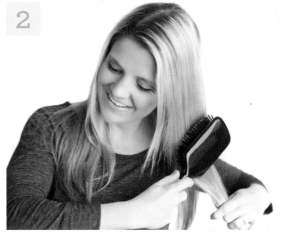

1 Start with dry hair.

2 Thoroughly brush through your hair with a paddle brush to gently remove any tangles.

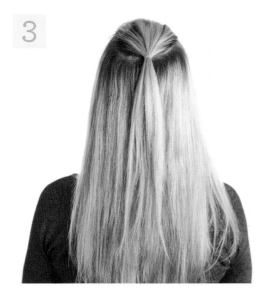

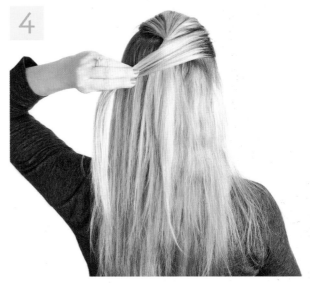

3 Using a rattail comb if necessary, part your hair from recession point to recession point in a slight U shape on the top of your head. Gather this section of hair and secure it with a clear elastic band.

4 Pick up a horizontal section of hair from the right side of your ponytail about 1 or 2 inches (2.5 to 5cm) wide. Cross that section over your center ponytail.

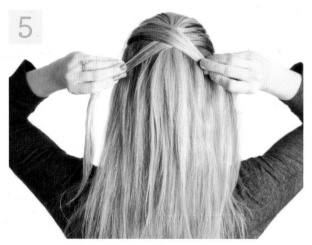

Pick up a horizontal section of hair from the left side of your ponytail about 1 or 2 inches (2.5 to 5cm) wide, and cross that piece over the center section.

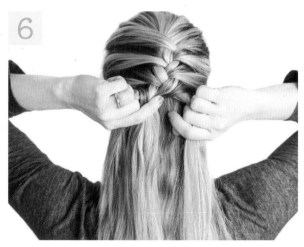

Continue picking up horizontal sections of hair from both sides, working the right section over the center section and then working the left section over the center as you move down the back of your head.

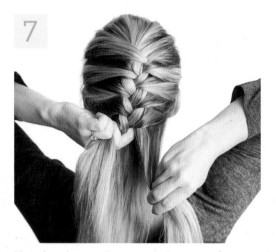

Keep braiding until you reach the nape of your neck and you have no more horizontal sections to pick up and add in.

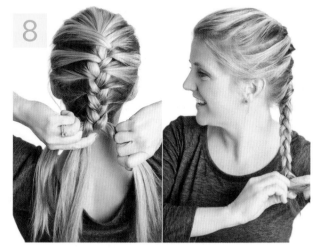

Continue braiding the rest of your hair to the ends. You can swing the braid around one of your shoulders to the front to make it easier on your arms as you finish the ends of the braid.

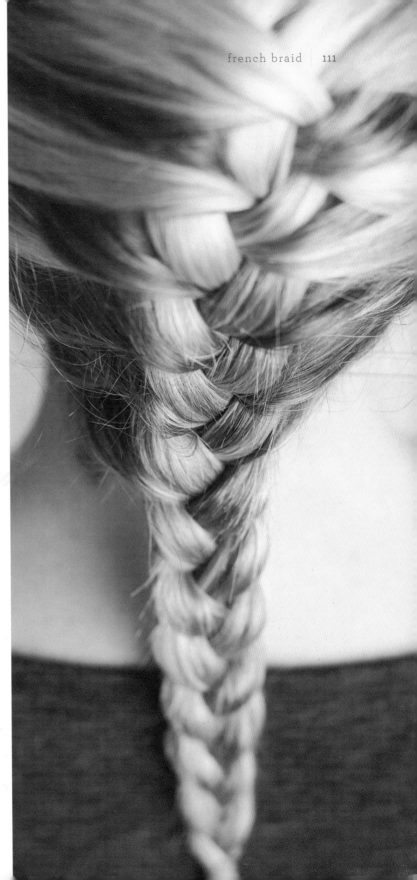

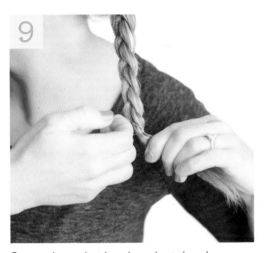

Secure the end with a clear elastic band.

If you want, you can cover the clear elastic band in the top section of your hair, or you can cut it with scissors for a more seamless look.

You also can pull out a few pieces of hair around your hairline for a slightly undone look.

Prairie Braid

This simple style is both bohemian and chic—think a modern take on the classic milkmaid up-do. If you're looking for an easy summer style to keep your hair up and out of your way, this one is for you. Wavy and straight strands will find this look most attainable.

TOOLS NEEDED

bobby pins

clear elastic bands

clips

defining paste (optional)

dry shampoo

rattail comb

teasing comb

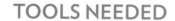

PREPPING YOUR HAIR | This style works best if you begin with hair that's been dried with a volumizing product for a little bounce on the top. If that's not an option, you can use dry shampoo to add texture to your hair so it will hold the style better.

1

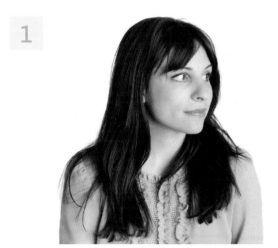

Start with dry hair.

2

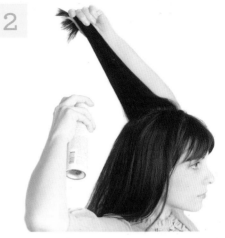

Lift sections of hair at your crown upward at a 90-degree angle from your head, and spray dry shampoo on the roots.

3

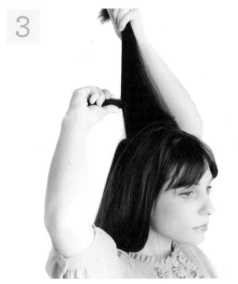

Gently tease your hair with a teasing comb for hold or added volume, whichever you prefer.

To tease correctly, hold a small section of hair upward at 90 degrees from your scalp and insert a teasing comb at about halfway down the hair shaft. Push the comb toward your head in a downward motion. Repeat this step until your crown area is lightly teased to your liking.

4

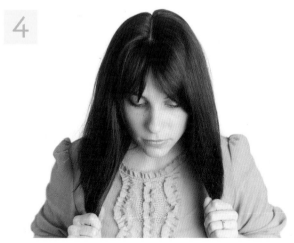

Using a rattail comb, part your hair down the center of your head so you have two equal sections.

5

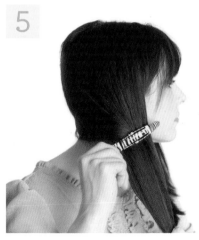

Clip the right side out of the way.

6

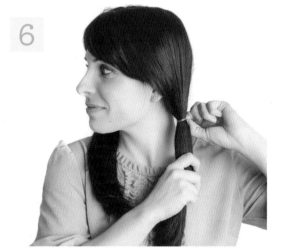

Gather the left side of your hair into a low ponytail and secure with a clear elastic band.

7

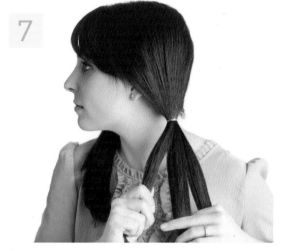

Divide that ponytail into three subsections.

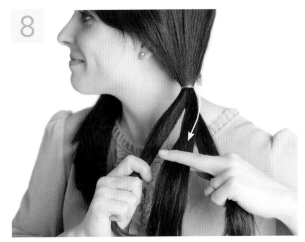

Braid the ponytail by crossing the right section over the center section.

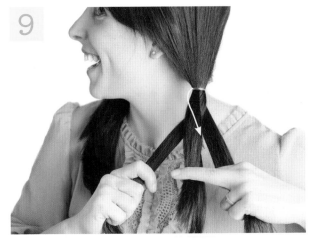

Cross the left section over the center section.

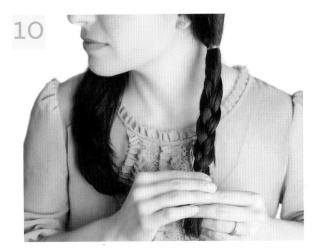

Continue crossing the right over the center and the left over the center until you reach the bottom of your ponytail.

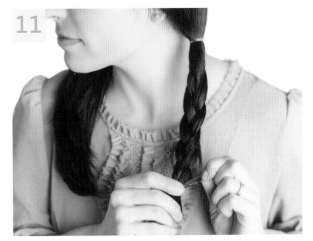

Secure the braid with a clear elastic band.

12

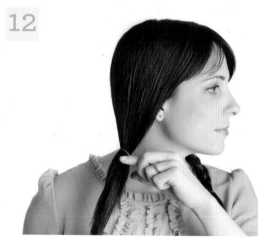

Unclip the right side of your hair, gather it into a low ponytail, and secure it with a clear elastic band.

13

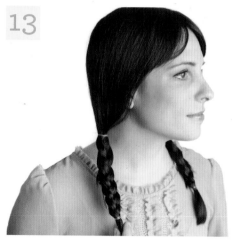

Repeat steps 7 through 10 for your right-side ponytail. You should now have two low braids.

14

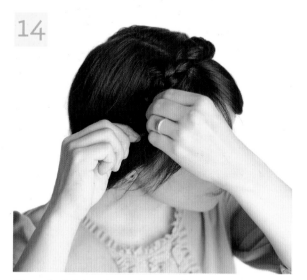

Cross the left braid over the top of your head about 1 or 2 inches (2.5 to 5cm) back from your hairline, and secure it with bobby pins.

15

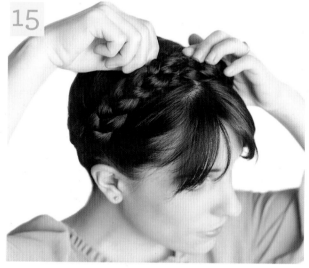

Cross the right braid over the top of your head, overlapping the left braid. Tuck the ends of the braids into each another so it looks like one continuous braid, and secure with bobby pins.

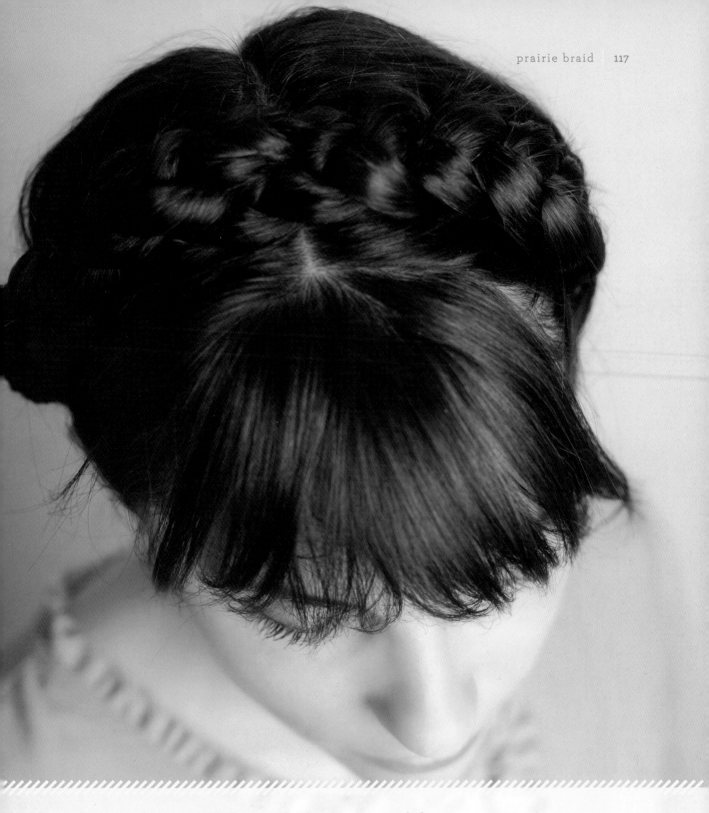

For a sleeker style or special occasion look, you can use defining paste to tame your tresses.

Inchworm Braid

This braid variation is great for keeping those shorter strands of hair at your front hairline under control. It's also a perfect—and stylish—alternative to pinning back your fringe or bangs, if you're trying to grow them out. All hair types can sport this look; however, those with curly hair may need to add a couple more products to tame their tresses before they're braided. You can wear this creative 'do casually when shopping with friends, or dress it up with a few curls for work or an evening out.

TOOLS NEEDED

clear elastic band
hairpins (optional)
medium-hold hairspray

rattail comb

PREPPING YOUR HAIR | If you have
curly hair, you'll want to use a moisturizing shampoo and conditioner first, before you apply any product. When your hair is towel dried, use an antifrizz or moisturizing serum to help combat frizz and flyaways. Then add a medium-hold mousse or styling lotion for hold. Next, either use a diffuser for added volume and curl, or let your curly strands dry naturally before beginning the braid. If you have naturally straight hair, you can smooth any unruly hairs with a flat iron before beginning the braid.

1

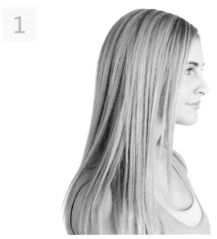

Start with dry hair that's straight, curly, or wavy, depending on how you'd like the majority of your hair to be styled.

2

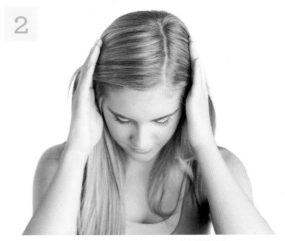

Using a rattail comb, cleanly part your hair either in the center of your head or on the side, whichever you feel most comfortable with.

3

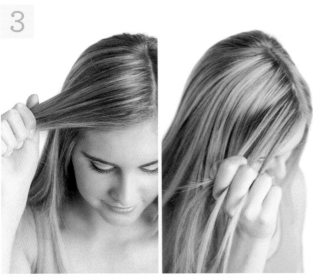

Gather a small section of hair toward your top hairline near your part, and divide it into three small subsections.

4

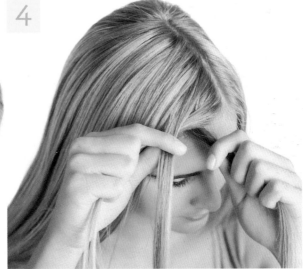

Overlap the first three sections as if you're starting a normal braid—cross the right section over the center section and then cross the left section over the center.

5

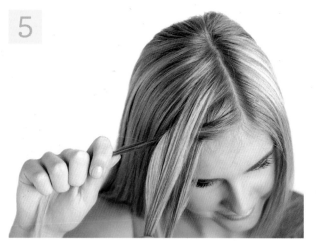

Pull additional hair from the top or part-side section, add it into the previous left subsection, and cross it all over the center.

6

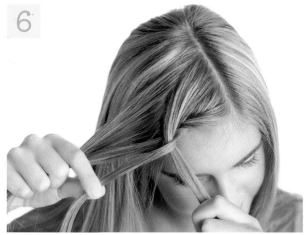

Cross the right piece over the center section, but do not add any additional hair to this section. Essentially, you're French braiding the top, part-side section and not the underneath section.

7

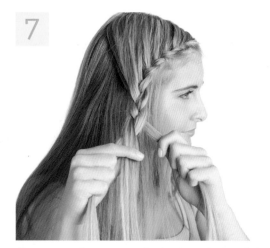

Continue with steps 5 and 6, keeping the braid close to your hairline to create the inchworm look. The sections on the right, or part side, of your hair that you're French braiding will keep getting longer the farther down you go on the braid. When you reach the bottom of your ear, you can stop French braiding and braid regularly until you reach the ends.

8

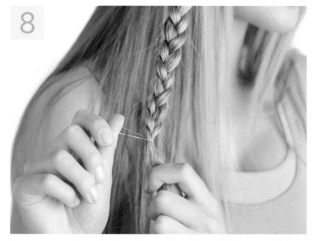

Secure your braid with a clear elastic band. You can add hairpins to secure any loose layers or pieces of hair that may have popped out while you were braiding.

9

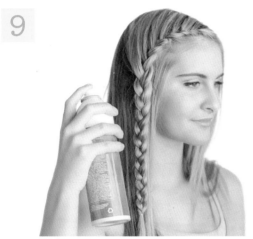

Finish with a medium-hold hairspray.

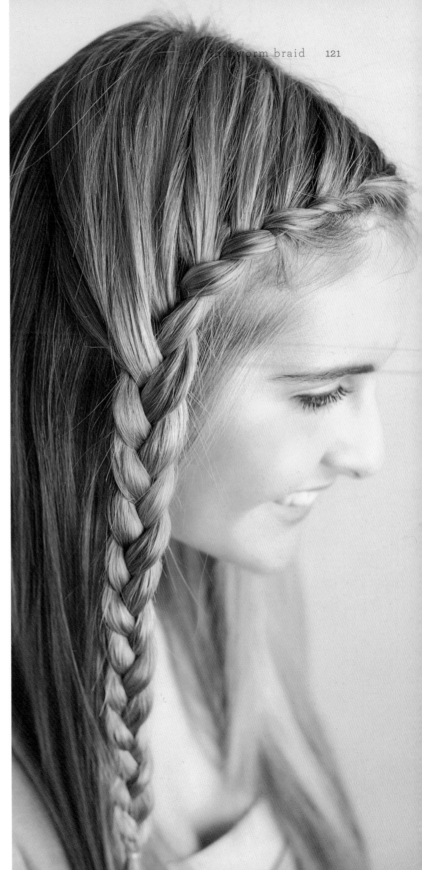

Braided Bun

This quick and easy bun has a bit more sass than the average bun. You can wear it for a Sunday stroll, tousle it a bit for a sensational runway look, or make it messy for a chic, ethereal feeling. All hair types can don this style.

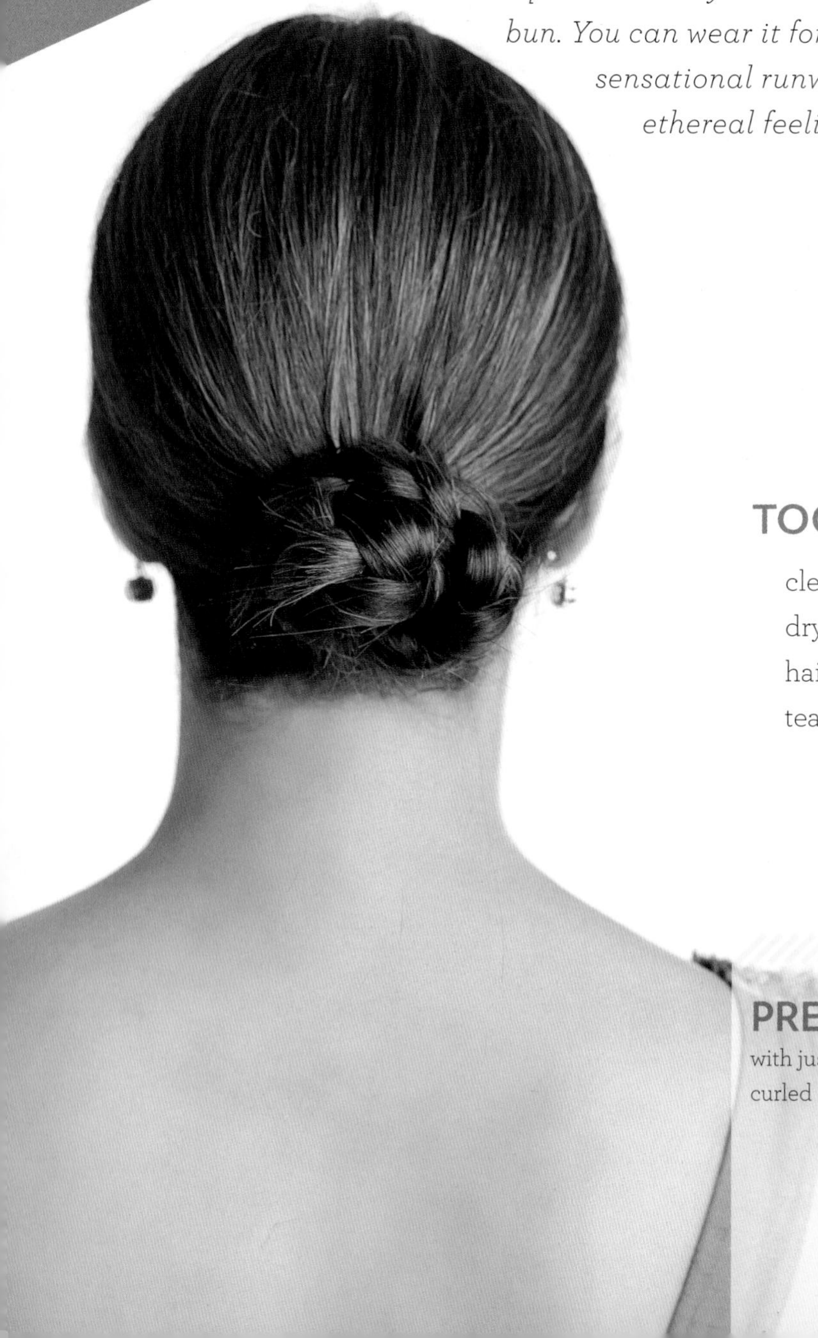

TOOLS NEEDED

clear elastic bands

dry shampoo

hairpins

teasing comb

PREPPING YOUR HAIR | You can start with just about any texture of hair for this style. Slightly curled or naturally textured hair will yield the best hold.

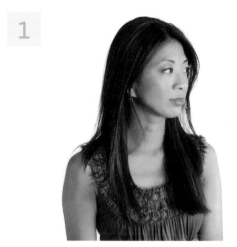

1

Start with dry hair.

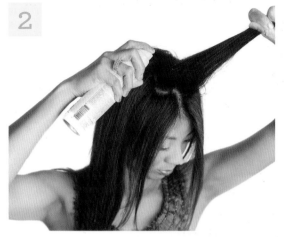

2

Grab a section of hair on your crown, and spray it with dry shampoo.

Some dry shampoos can leave a chalky residue in your hair. You might want to sample a few until you find one you like.

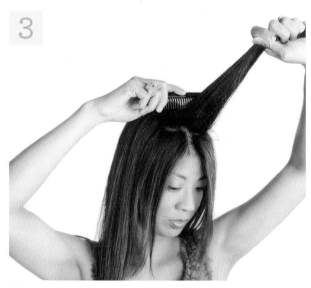

3

Using a teasing comb, tease your crown area for additional texture.

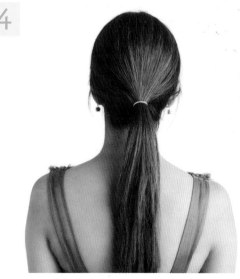

4

Gather your hair into either a high or low ponytail, depending on your desired look.

5

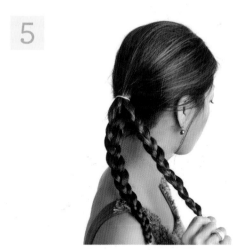

Divide your ponytail into two sections. Braid each section separately, and secure the ends with clear elastic bands.

6

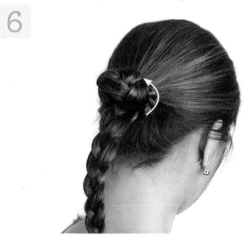

Twist one braid around the front part of the ponytail, over the clear elastic band, and secure it with hairpins.

7

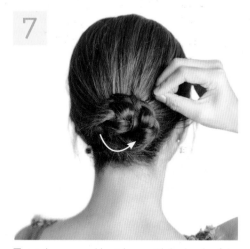

Twist the second braid around the back of the ponytail to complete the bun, and secure it with hairpins. Tuck in any additional hairs that are poking out with hairpins as well.

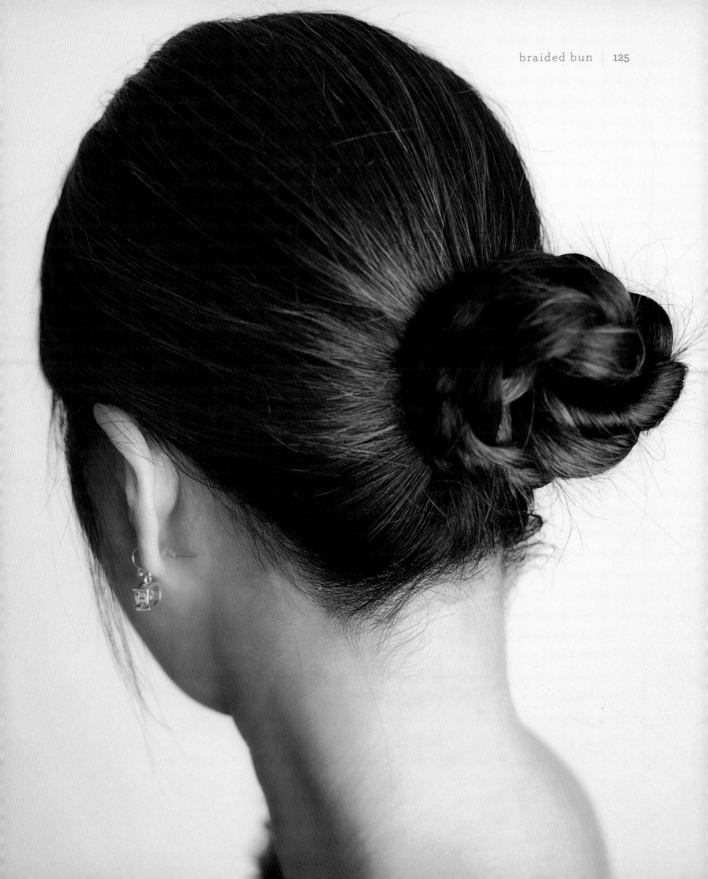

Fishtail

The braid is a classic that never goes out of style. This fresh new version of the classic braid is making a real splash at award shows, and it's simple enough you can do it at home, too. Wear it to the office, to school, or while running errands. It's a perfect style if you're on the go because it keeps those stray hairs out of your face. You can create a polished version for a special night out or a more casual tail with roughed-up texture and tendrils flowing naturally near your face. All textures work well with this fun style.

TOOLS NEEDED

clear elastic bands
rattail comb
volumizing powder

PREPPING YOUR HAIR | You can start with any texture of hair here. For an undone look, go with a messier texture and add a spray wax or sea-salt spray. Or you can curl your hair first with a large-barrel curling iron and then mold your curly locks into the fishtail for a more polished, sophisticated look.

1

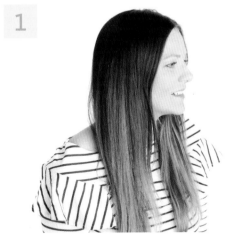

Start with dry hair.

2

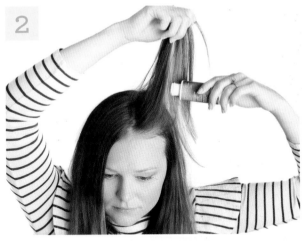

Working in your crown area, sprinkle your roots all over the top of your head with a volumizing powder.

3

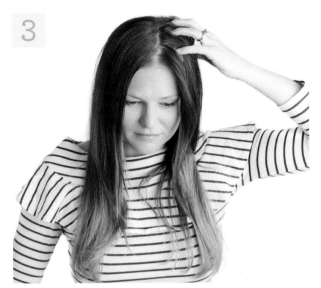

Push your fingers onto your hair to your scalp where you sprinkled the powder, and rub gently back and forth with your fingertips. This helps activate the powder for extra lift.

4

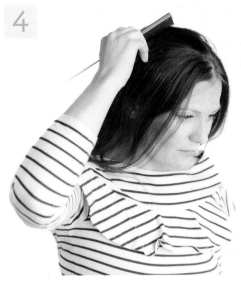

Using your rattail comb, lightly comb over your volumized area.

5

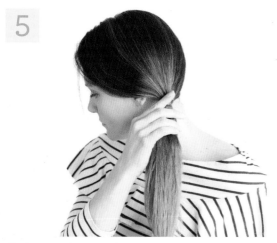

Gather your hair in either a low ponytail or low side ponytail, and secure with a clear elastic band.

6

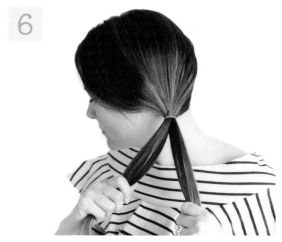

Divide your ponytail into two equal sections.

7

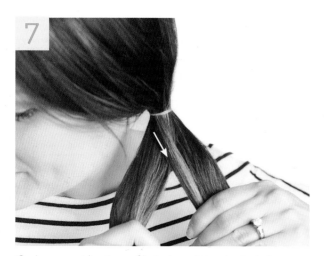

Grab an outside piece of hair about $\frac{1}{8}$ to $\frac{1}{4}$ inch (3mm to .5cm) wide, pull it over the left section, and feed it into the right section. Be sure to keep your ponytail in two separate sections.

8

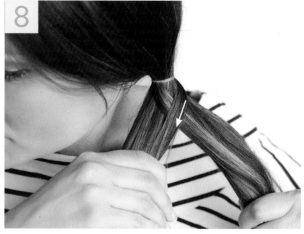

Grab another outside piece of hair about $\frac{1}{8}$ to $\frac{1}{4}$ inch (3mm to .5cm) wide, this time on the right side. Pull it over your right side, and feed it into the left section.

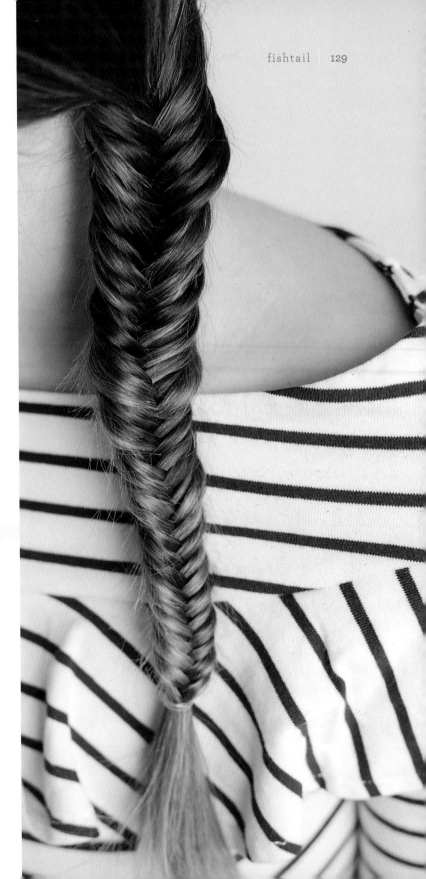

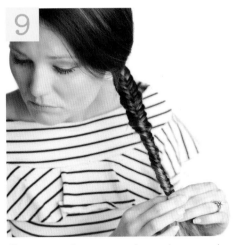

9

Continue with steps 7 and 8 until you reach the bottom of your ponytail. Leave about 1 or 2 inches (2.5 to 5cm) unbraided at the bottom, and secure the ends with another clear elastic band.

To create a more natural flow from your hair into the fishtail, you can cut the first clear elastic you put in at the start of your tail.

Bombshell Curls

You'll feel like the life of the party with this gorgeous, classic style. A look this glamorous is best for a night on the town, your best friend's wedding, or a special event that's red carpet worthy. Although this is one of the more time-consuming styles in the book because of all the sectioning and clipping you do before you curl your hair, the end result is totally worth it! All hair types and textures can try this look.

TOOLS NEEDED

boar bristle brush

curling iron with a 1¼-inch (3cm) barrel

duckbill clips

long metal clips

medium-hold hairspray

rattail comb

volumizing mousse or light-hold gel

PREPPING YOUR HAIR | Although this style works in any hair, if you have curly hair, blow it out smooth before attempting this look.

1

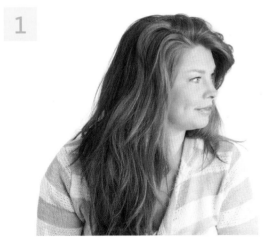

Start with dry hair.

2

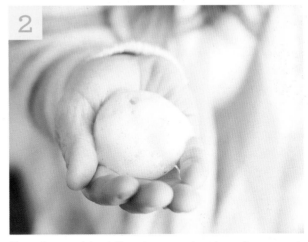

For volume, add a dollop about 3 inches (7.5cm) in diameter of a light-hold product such as a volumizing mousse or light-hold gel throughout your tresses.

3

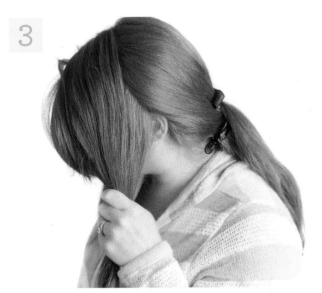

Using a rattail comb, divide your hair into two sections, from ear to ear.

4

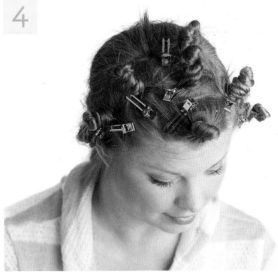

Divide your front section of hair into six or seven 2-inch (5cm) horizontal subsections. If you have bangs, you can section them out separately. Twist each section of hair as you separate it, and pin it with a duckbill clip to secure it out of the way. Split the back section into horizontal 2-inch (5cm) sections as well.

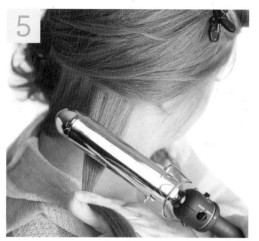

Starting at the bottom of your head and using a 1 ¼-inch (3cm) curling iron, unclip and wrap a section of hair around the curling iron that's pointed down. Push on the base of your hair to heat it and push it how you want it to lay.

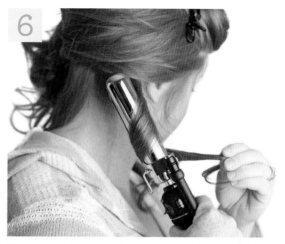

Wrap your hair around the iron so it's flat and isn't twisted against the barrel.

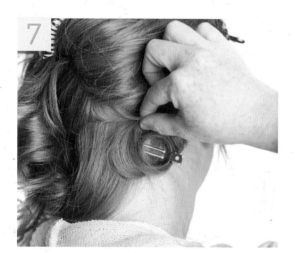

Remove the curling iron, and pin the curl with a duckbill clip to set. Continue unpinning and wrapping sections of hair around the iron, alternating directions for each curl. (Curl one section forward and the next backward.)

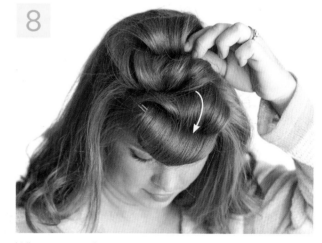

When you reach your top two sections of hair, curl them forward and not directly on top of your head. You don't want a lot of volume at your crown.

9

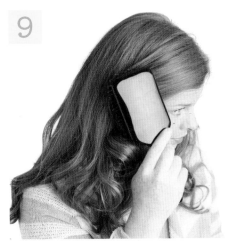

When all your hair is curled, cooled, and set, remove the duckbill clips and gently brush your hair with a boar bristle brush.

10

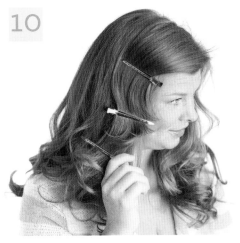

If you need to, you can insert a few longer metal clips to help reshape your style to be sure the curls curl the way you want them to and ensure the waves will stay. Let your clipped curls rest for a bit before removing the clips. Finish with a medium-hold hairspray.

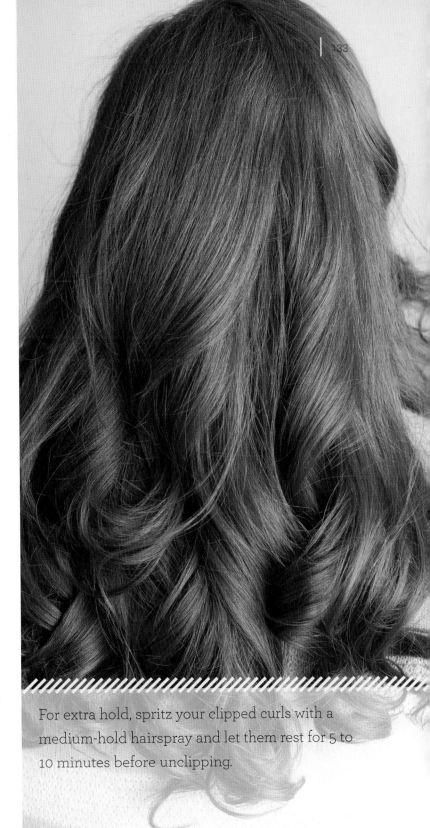

For extra hold, spritz your clipped curls with a medium-hold hairspray and let them rest for 5 to 10 minutes before unclipping.

Mermaid Waves

Many little girls dream of having hair as long and pretty as a mermaid. Well, now your dreams can come true, thanks to your handy curling iron or wand. Although these swirls are more refined and don't look like you just came from a day at the beach, they can be low-key enough to wear to your neighbor's summer barbecue. Mermaid Waves are also a great foundation for fancier styles such as a low-slung fishtail, braid, or twist. All textures of hair can conquer this look.

TOOLS NEEDED

blow-dryer

clips

concentrator

curling iron or wand with a $3/4$- to $1^1/_2$-inch (2 to 3.75cm) barrel, depending on how tight you want your waves

defining paste

paddle brush

sea-salt spray

volumizing spray

1

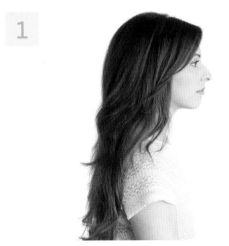

Start with dry hair with some natural texture.

2

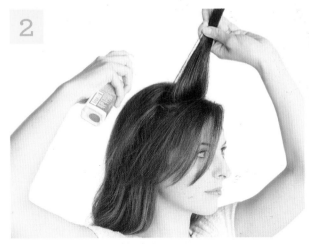

Raise small sections of hair in your crown area, and spritz with volumizing spray at the roots.

3

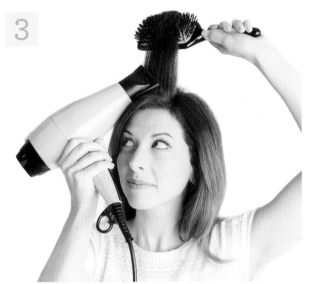

Use a paddle brush to lift your hair at 90 degrees from your head. While the ends of your strands are resting in the paddle brush, use a blow-dryer fitted with a concentrator to blow your hair from the roots to the ends. The combination of the volumizing spray and the blow-dryer on your dry hair creates volume and lift at your crown. Continue all over the crown area of your head.

4

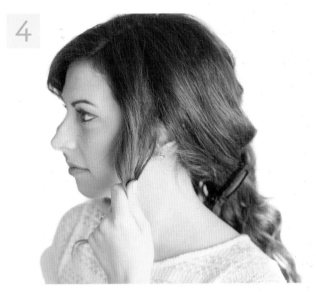

Separate a vertical section of hair close to your face, and clip the rest of your hair out of your way.

5

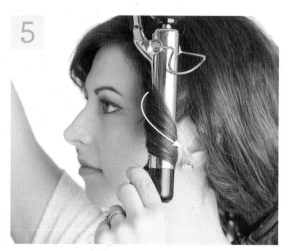

Using a curling iron or wand with a $^3/_4$- to $1^1/_2$-inch (2 to 3.75cm) barrel, tilt the iron upside down so the hot part is pointed downward. Wrap your vertical section of hair around the iron so it goes away from your face, leaving about 1 or 2 inches (2.5 to 5cm) at the bottom uncurled.

6

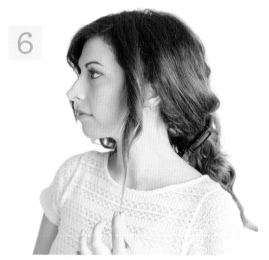

Drop your hair from the curling iron, and tug on the ends to loosen the tendril. Separate another vertical section of hair next to the first, clip the rest of your hair back, and repeat curling until you reach the back middle area of your head.

7

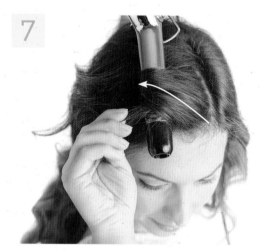

Move to the opposite side of your face, section out another vertical section of hair, and clip the rest of your uncurled hair out of the way. Repeat steps 5 and 6 until you reach the back middle part of your hair. All of your hair should be curled now.

8

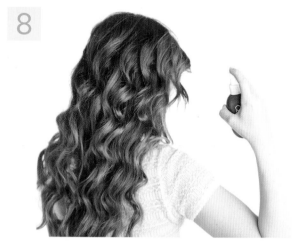

Lightly spritz your waves with sea-salt spray.

9

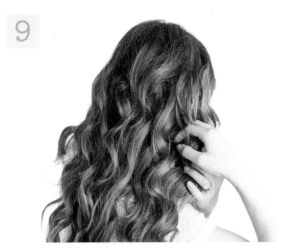

Gently separate your waves with your fingers.

10

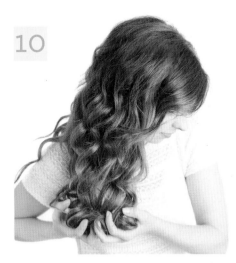

Disperse about a pea-size dollop of defining paste into your palms, and rub your palms together until you no longer see the product. Scrunch the paste into your waves.

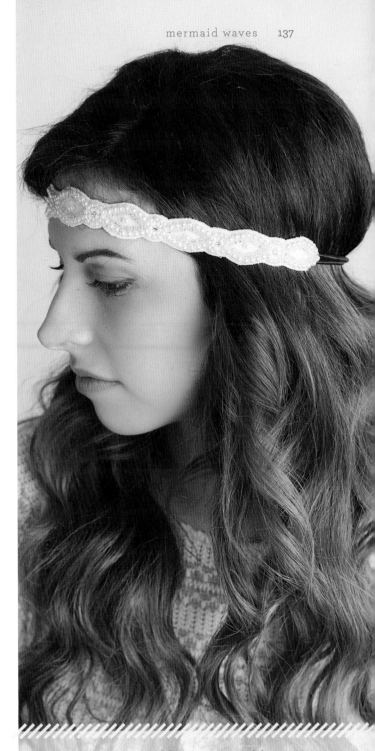

For some extra sparkle, you can add a beaded headband.

Top Knot

Some days you probably don't want to spend a large amount of time on your hair, but you still want it to look polished. On days like this, the Top Knot is your new go-to 'do. This also is a great way to disguise second- or third-day hair if you don't wash your locks every day (washing your hair every day isn't always ideal) and is a great extender for a blowout. All textures can wear this style, but straight- and wavy-haired gals fare best.

TOOLS NEEDED

bobby pins (optional)

clear elastic band

hairpins

medium- to firm-hold hairspray

root-lifting foam

smoothing serum or paste (optional)

teasing comb

PREPPING YOUR HAIR | You can start
with any kind of texture to your hair. But for best results, if you have super silky strands, you'll want to give them some texture so they'll better stay in the bun.

1

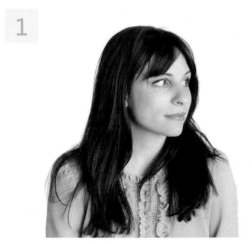

Start with dry hair.

2

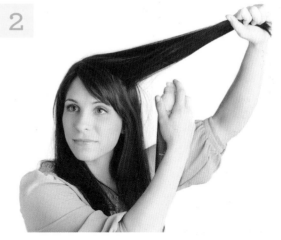

Rough up the texture at your roots by applying a root-lifting foam to your scalp in your crown area. Do this by parting out long horizontal sections and placing the foam directly on your scalp.

3

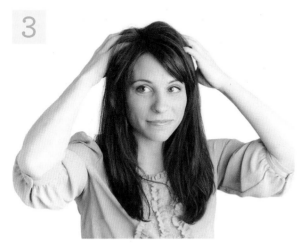

Rub the foam into your roots with your fingertips to create even more texture.

4

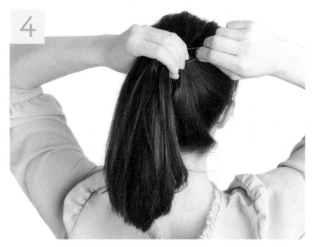

Gather your hair into a high ponytail with your hands. Be sure your pony is free of bumps or knots. You want your hair to look uniform, but not slick and smooth. Secure the pony with a clear elastic band.

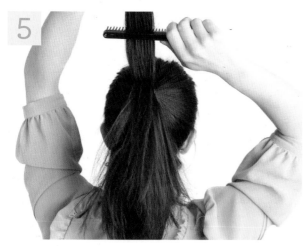

Tease your ponytail thoroughly using a your teasing comb. This style won't hold unless your hair has plenty of texture.

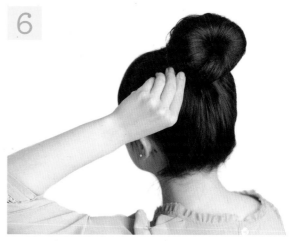

Wrap the ponytail around the front of your head in a loose manner to begin forming the knot.

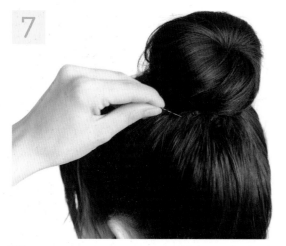

Continue wrapping your pony and forming the knot until you can tuck the ends underneath the knot. Secure the knot with hairpins at first, and if needed, add bobby pins for extra stability.

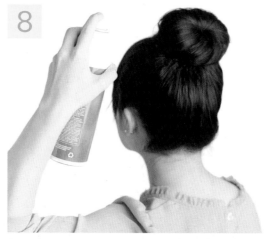

Set your hair with a medium- to firm-hold hairspray. If you have textured or damaged hair, you can use a smoothing serum or paste to help tame frizz and flyaways along the base of your ponytail.

Make this style look ultramodern by placing a bow or decorative barrette directly below the knot on the underside.

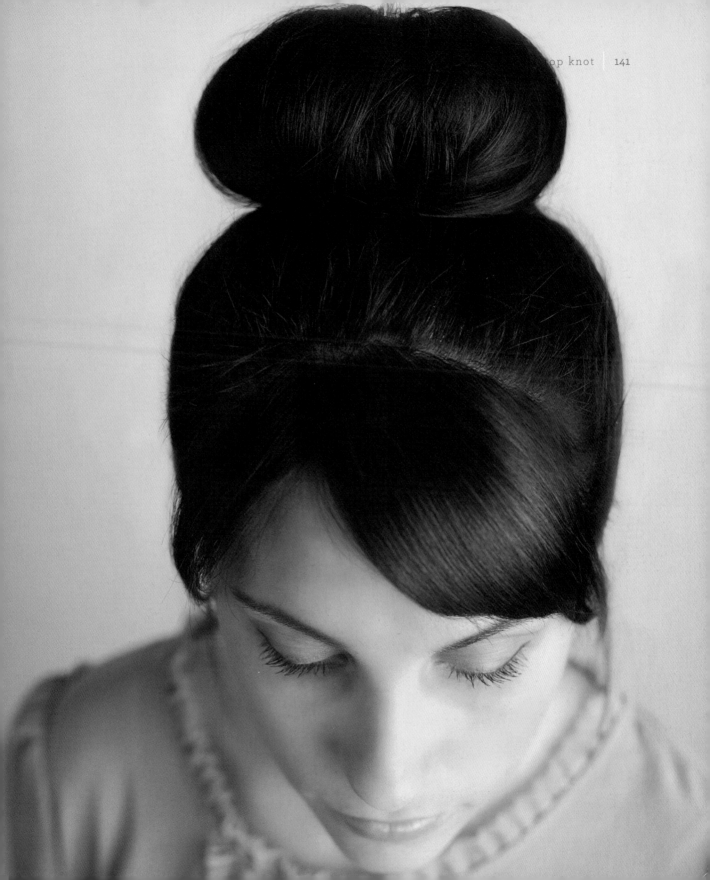

High Roller

Want big, luscious curls but don't want to spend a lot of time getting them? Your hot rollers can help! Hot rollers aren't as commonly used as they used to be, but when used correctly, they're a simple, time-saving way to get bouncy, voluminous locks. Mothers and multi-taskers will appreciate the ease of putting in the curlers and then being able to do other things while they cool and curl your hair. All hair types can use hot rollers. Be sure your rollers are hot and ready to go before you put them in your hair!

TOOLS NEEDED

boar bristle brush

clips

flat metal clips

hot rollers

light-hold curl-enhancing mousse

light-hold or working hairspray

PREPPING YOUR HAIR | If you have naturally curly hair, especially if it's tightly curled, you might want to blow it out straight first before attempting this look. You'll have better luck getting smoother curls if you start with straighter hair.

1

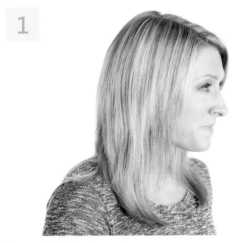

Start with dry hair.

2

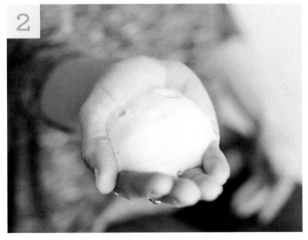

Dispense a small amount of light-hold curl-enhancing mousse into your hands, approximately a 3-inch (7.5cm) palmful for each side of your hair. You want to use just enough to allow for extra hold.

3

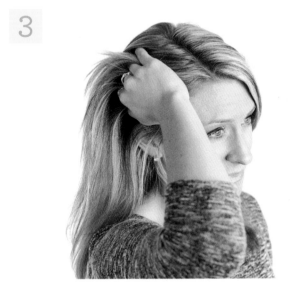

Apply the mousse to your hair, working it through to the ends.

4

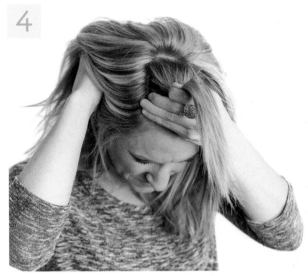

Section out a strip of hair down the center of your head (like a Mohawk), no wider than the size of a roller. Clip the rest of your hair out of the way.

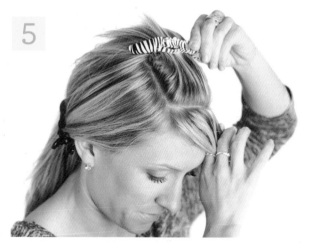

5

With your Mohawk section parted out, pull out a subsection the length and width of one roller at your hairline. Clip the rest of the Mohawk section out of the way.

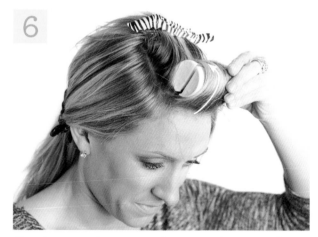

6

Overdirect your hair past 90 degrees, and insert a roller into your hair, rolling backward away from your face. Be sure all of the section of hair is pulled seamlessly into the roller to avoid any kinks.

Overdirecting your hair past 90 degrees adds the most volume to the finished style. Be sure to direct each section as you roll for maximum body.

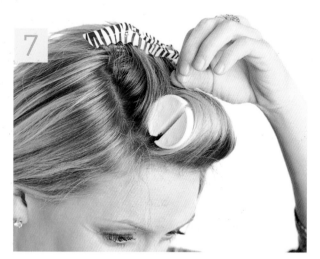

7

When the roller has reached your scalp and you're ready to secure it, insert a flat metal clip at the base of your hair, ensuring that you've gotten the hair in the roller and the hair at the base to hold it in place while it cools. If needed, insert another clip on the other side.

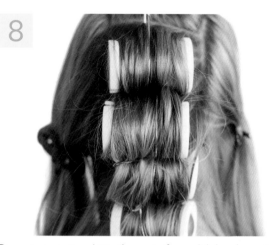

8

Repeat steps 6 and 7 in the rest of your Mohawk section all the way down your head to the nape of your neck. Then move to the sides of your head and repeat, sectioning out your hair the width of one roller at a time, until your entire head is full of rollers.

9

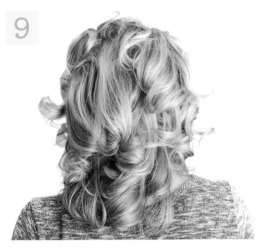

Let the rollers cool for about 20 to 25 minutes. When they're cool, gently take them all out.

10

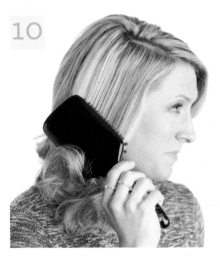

Comb through your hair with your fingers for a tousled, bouncy look, or use a boar bristle brush for a smooth and polished style. Finish with a light-hold or working hairspray so your hair can still move freely.

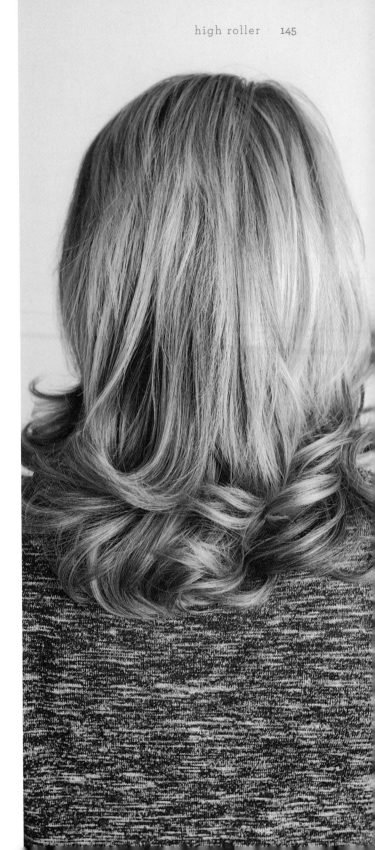

Polished Pony

The traditional ponytail is quite effortless and takes little time to achieve. However, with a simple twist on the basic pony, your tresses can look polished enough to wear to a business meeting or glam enough to wear with a party dress. The Polished Pony starts with hair that's been carefully straightened with a flat iron and then pulled into a strategic ponytail. The twist comes when you wrap a piece of hair around the clear elastic band for a chic update. Although this style hardly takes any time at all, it looks like you put a bit of work into it. All hair textures can achieve this look.

TOOLS NEEDED

bobby pin

clear elastic bands

clips

defining paste

flat iron

hairspray

heat-resistant comb

PREPPING YOUR HAIR | The key to
achieving the "polished" part of this hairstyle is smoothly straightening your hair. If you have very tight curly hair, you might want to blow it out before you begin straightening.

1

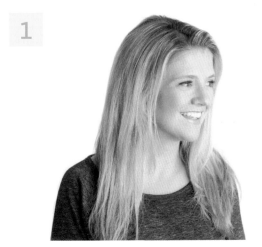

Start with dry hair.

2

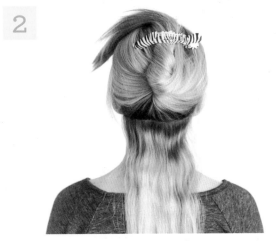

Starting at the nape of your neck, section off an area of hair approximately 2 inches (5cm) up from your hairline, and clip the rest of your hair up and out of the way.

3

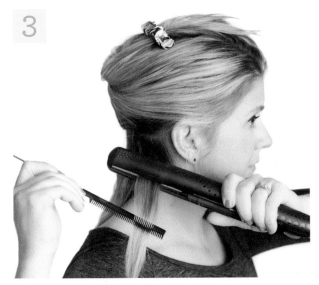

Place a heat-resistant comb underneath a 2×2-inch (5×5cm) subsection of hair at a 45-degree angle. Place a flat iron above the heat-resistant comb, and clamp down. Iron your hair, traveling approximately 1 inch (2.5cm) per second down the hair shaft, until that subsection is straight. Repeat until you finish the section of hair at the nape of your neck.

Resist the urge to flat iron your hair too much. You should only need to go over each section of your hair one or two times with the flat iron to successfully straighten it. If you iron it any more than that, you're likely to end up with limp, lifeless locks.

4

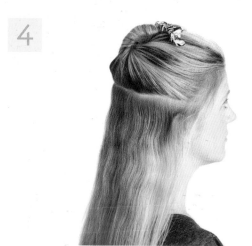

Section off another 2-inch (5cm) area of hair just above the last, and repeat step 3 until that entire area is straight. Continue straightening 2-inch (5cm) sections of hair all around and over your head until all your hair has been flat ironed.

When you reach the crown of your head, hold the comb and flat iron at a 90-degree angle to your scalp instead of 45 degrees like you used elsewhere. This helps you achieve maximum volume in your crown. And to add even more volume, you can tease your crown with a teasing comb.

5

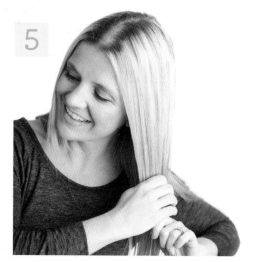

Distribute a small amount of defining paste in your palm, and rub your palms together. Distribute the defining paste throughout your hair for light hold when styling your ponytail.

6

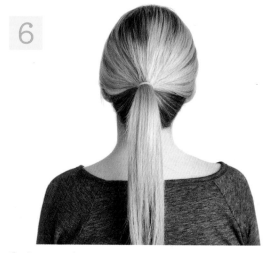

Gather your hair into a medium to low ponytail, and secure with a clear elastic band.

7

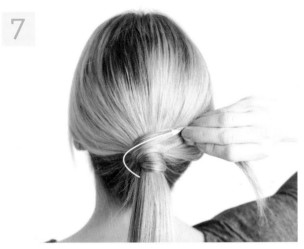

Take a small piece of hair from the bottom side of the ponytail you just created, and wrap it around the clear elastic band.

8

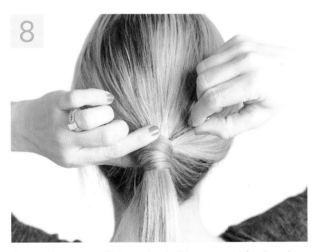

Secure the piece of hair with a bobby pin, and finish with a light coat of hairspray.

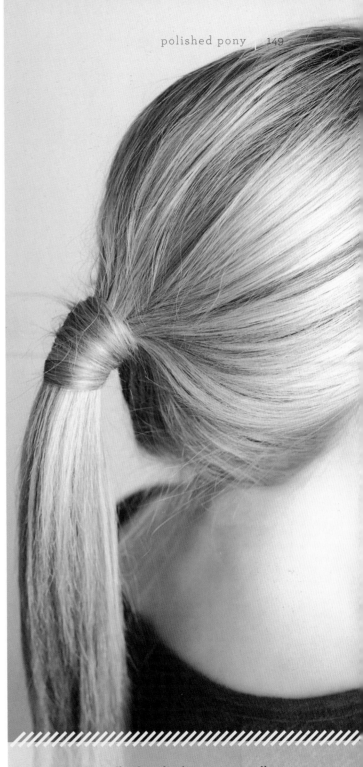

For a pretty yet effortless look, you can pull out a few loose layers or pieces around your face.

Knot Your Basic Bun

The bun has been around for ages and can be dressed up or dressed down easily for different looks. This version can go either dressy or casual, too, but whichever way you take it, it's sure to be eye-catching. In Knot Your Basic Bun, you literally tie your hair in knots. The look is quite unique and very manageable for all hair types and textures, even extremely curly hair.

TOOLS NEEDED

bobby pins and/or hairpins

clear elastic band

hairspray

teasing comb (optional)

volumizing mousse

PREPPING YOUR HAIR | For this style, you can start with hair that's been dried naturally, blown out straight and sleek, or anything in between.

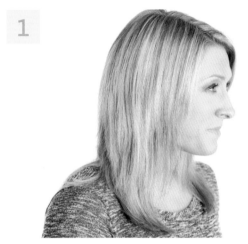

1

Start with dry hair.

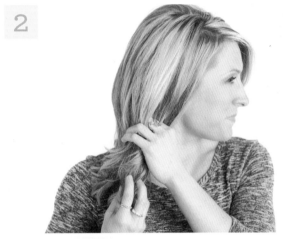

2

Disperse a 3-inch (7.5 cm) dollop of volumizing mousse about the size of your palm into your hand. Smooth the mousse into your hands a bit, and apply it to the middle and ends of your hair for additional hold.

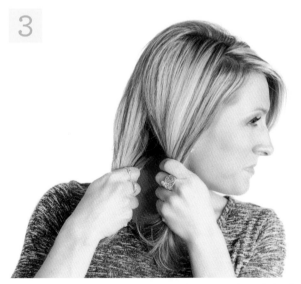

3

Gather your hair low on one side of your head, and divide it into two equal sections.

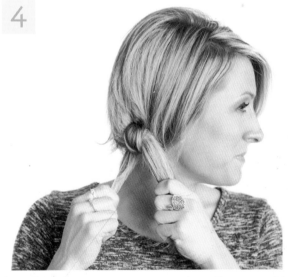

4

Literally tie these two sections into a knot, like you would tie the first knot when tying your shoes. Keep the knot very close to your head, low and at the base.

5

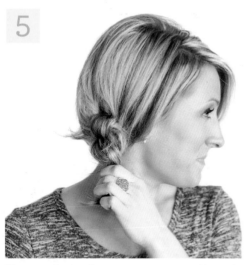

Keeping the first knot taut, tie a second knot the same way just below it.

6

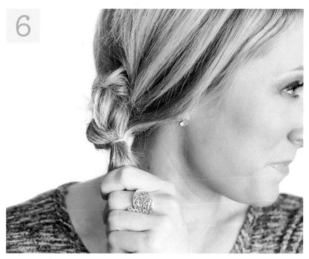

Combine the two tails into one section. Continue to keep the two knots tight at the base of your scalp, and secure the ends of your hair into ponytail with a clear elastic band right under the second knot.

7

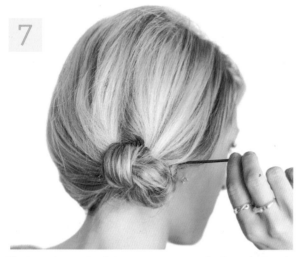

Tuck up the ends of the pony to create the bun, and push the elastic band up into the second knot to hide it. You can loosen the bottom strand of the second knot just a bit to cover the elastic band a little better. Use bobby pins and/ or hairpins to secure the ends.

8

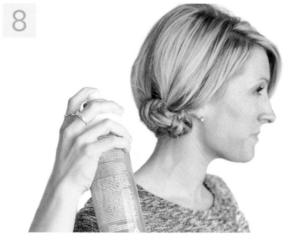

Finish with a veil of hairspray.

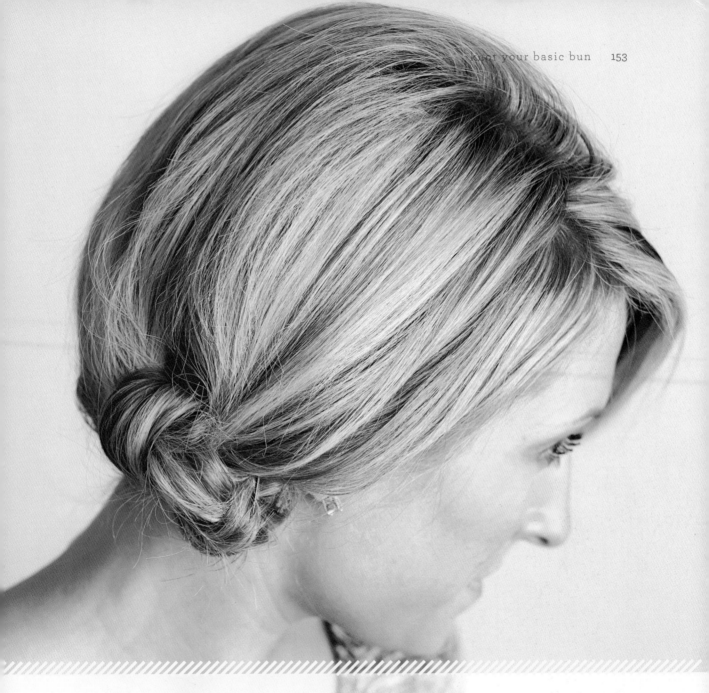

If you have short layers, you might need to add bobby pins or hairpins to the side of your hair opposite your knot to ensure you don't have any flyaways.

If your hair is longer, rather than tucking the ends up into a bun in step 7, you can use a teasing comb to add a little texture to the ends of your ponytail and leave it down. You also can add another palmful of mousse to your pony for increased texture.

Crown and Glory

Picture yourself front and center at a summer music festival or picnicking in the park with these lovely plaits. This urban hippie version of half-up hair looks like you've put effort into your look yet not stood in the mirror for hours adjusting every hair until each strand is perfect. This no-fuss fashion is good for most any hair type.

TOOLS NEEDED

bobby pins and/or hairpins

clear elastic band

clips

curling iron or wand with a 1¼-inch (3cm) barrel

defining paste

PREPPING YOUR HAIR | Nearly any hair type works with this 'do, but the more texture you naturally have in your hair, the better your finished Crown and Glory will look.

1

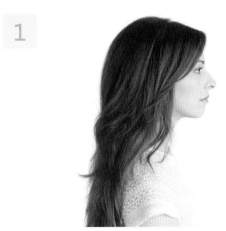

Start with dry hair.

2

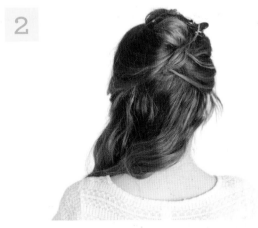

Separate your hair into two equal sections, one on top and one on bottom, parting from the top of one ear around the back of your head to the top of the other ear. Clip up the top section.

3

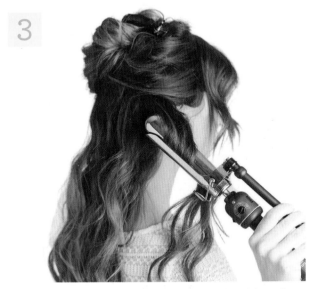

Use a curling iron or wand with a 1¼-inch (3cm) barrel to add texture to your hair. Hold a 2-inch-wide (5cm-wide) section of hair closest to your face outward at a 45-degree angle from your head. Insert this section of hair into your open curling iron with the clamp facing forward. You'll want to close the curling iron in the middle of the strand.

4

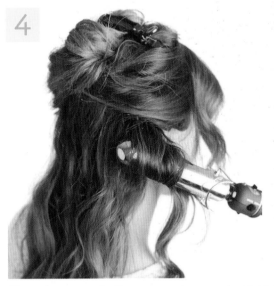

Close the iron, and roll it up toward your scalp. Hold there for 2 or 3 seconds. Continue curling until your entire head is curled.

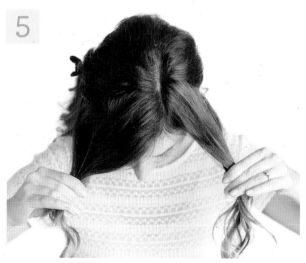

Part out a 2-inch (5cm) section of hair along your front hairline, and clip this section out of the way. Give yourself a center or side part.

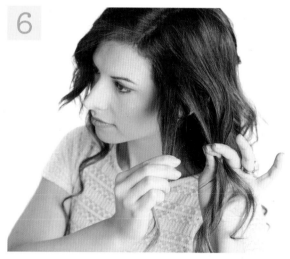

Divide the section on one side of your part into three subsections.

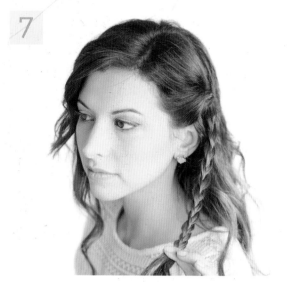

Either French braid for a couple strands and then transition to a regular braid, or do a regular braid from the start. When you've finished the braid, secure it with a clear elastic band.

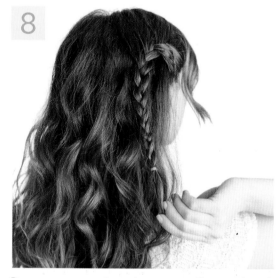

Repeat steps 6 and 7 in the section of hair on the other side of your part. You should now have two braids.

9

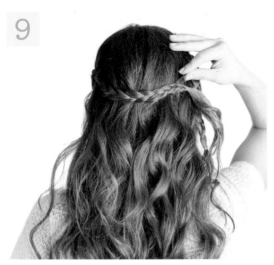

Swing the right braid behind your head a little loosely, and use hairpins or bobby pins to secure it.

10

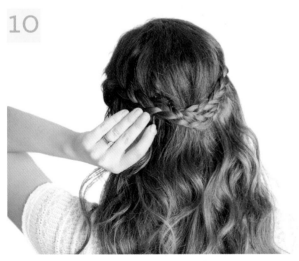

Swing the other braid behind your head, over the first braid, and tuck it into the other braid. Try to hide the elastic band under the other braid, and insert bobby pins where necessary to anchor the braids to your head so they don't move.

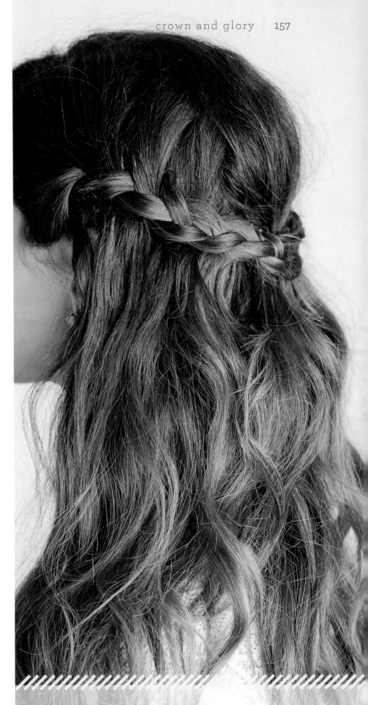

For more texture, use a dab of defining paste on your fingertips to pull out and style some strands around your bangs.

Festival Braided Knot

This organic version of the braid is showing up everywhere from summer music festivals to the red carpet. Let your inner flower child out to play, and give this fun style a try. It's made of two French braids leading down into a ponytail, with random tendrils falling out of the style to create an earthy, undone look.

TOOLS NEEDED

bobby pin

clear elastic band

clips

dry shampoo

maximum-hold hairspray (optional)

spray wax (optional)

teasing comb

PREPPING YOUR HAIR | Let your hair dry naturally if you have wavy or curly hair. If you have straight hair, add some texture with a curling iron or wand before attempting this 'do.

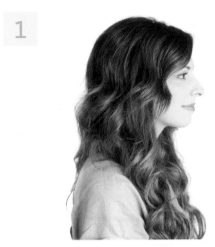

1

Start with dry hair.

2

Spray a couple shots of dry shampoo on your roots in your crown area for added volume.

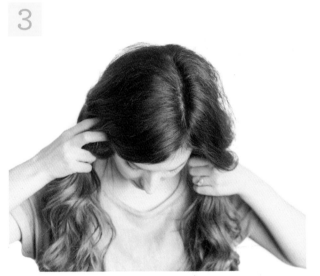

3

Part your hair down the center or on the side so you have two mostly equal-size sections.

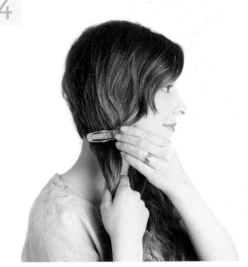

4

Clip the right side of your hair out of the way so you can start to braid the left section.

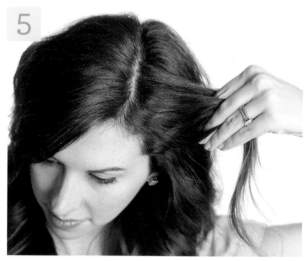

Starting on the top of your left section, gather three pieces of hair.

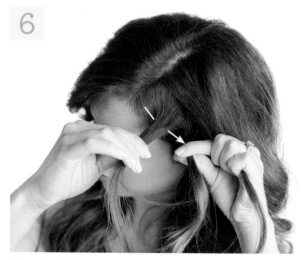

Cross the left section *under* the center section.

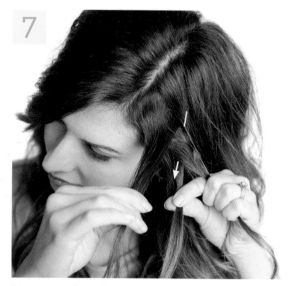

Next, cross the right section under the center section.

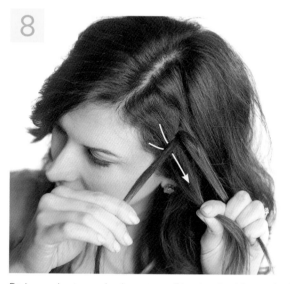

Pick up a horizontal subsection of hair and add it to the left side section. Cross your newly larger left side under the center.

9

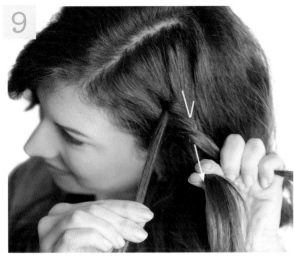

Pick up another horizontal subsection of hair and feed it into the right side section. Cross your newly larger right side under the center.

10

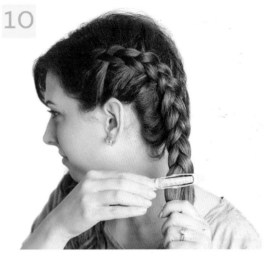

Continue with steps 8 and 9 until you reach the nape of your neck. Clip your braid so it doesn't unravel.

11

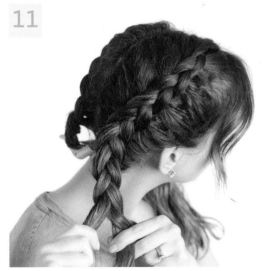

Repeat the inverted French braid on the right section of your hair.

12

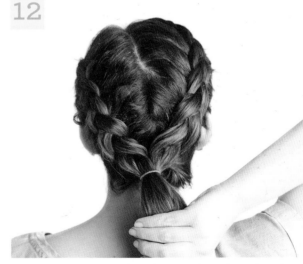

When you reach the nape of your neck on the right side, unclip the left side braid, combine the two braids, and secure them with a clear elastic band.

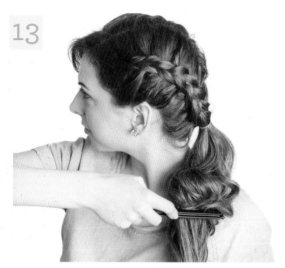

13

Add more texture to your ponytail by teasing small sections upward using a teasing comb. Tease until your entire ponytail has lots of texture.

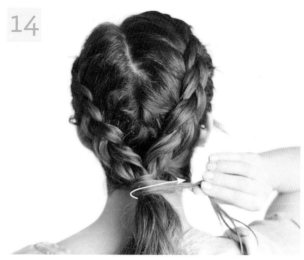

14

Pull out a piece of hair from under your ponytail, wrap it around the elastic band, and secure it with a bobby pin under your ponytail.

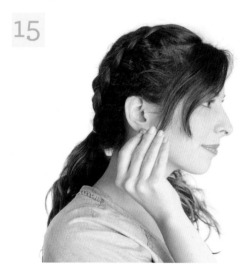

15

Leave out your bangs and any shorter layers to delicately frame your face. Remember, you don't want every hair to be in its perfect place.

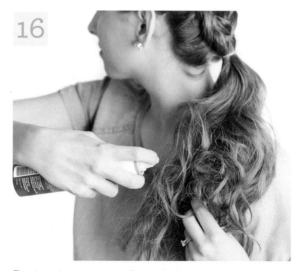

16

Finish with a spray wax for added texture and volume if you have fine hair, or you can opt for a hairspray with maximum hold. Spray all over your ponytail, or just upward on the ends.

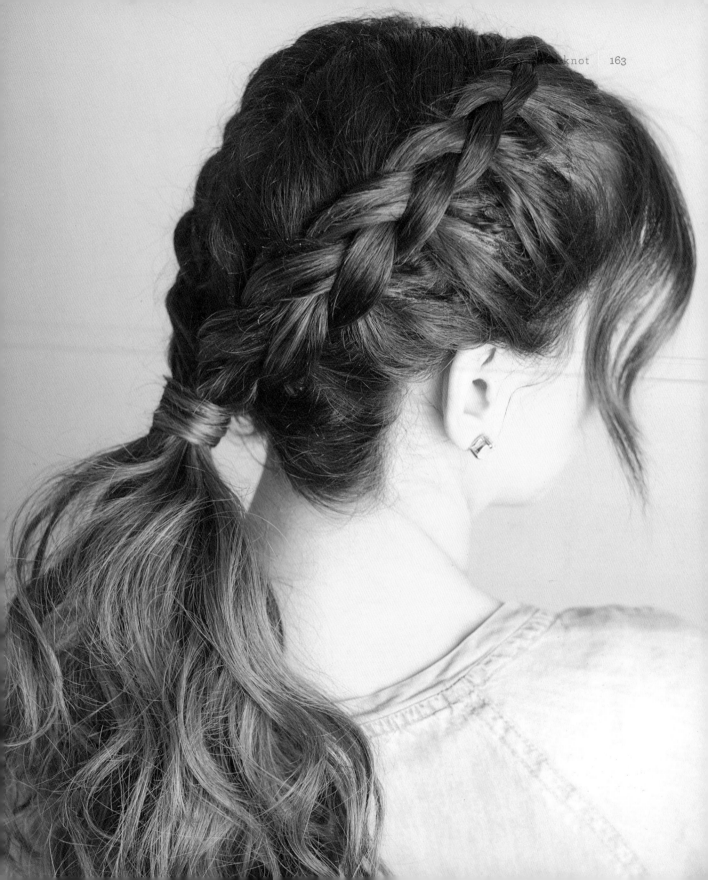

Bear Claw Ponytail

At first sight, this twisted hairstyle brings to mind the bear claw doughnut, hence the name. Although this hairstyle isn't sticky like its pastry namesake, it is sweet enough to satisfy your craving for a fresh new look. Picture yourself out strolling through your local farmers' market on a Saturday morning or rocking out to your favorite band at an outdoor summer concert sporting this low-slung, side twist. All hair types can twist into this style.

TOOLS NEEDED

bobby pin (optional)
clear elastic band
clips
hairpins (optional)
rattail comb

PREPPING YOUR HAIR | For slight
volume, apply a few sprays of dry shampoo at your roots. For lots more volume, use a teasing comb to tease your crown.

1

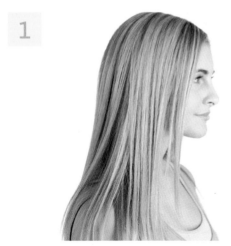

Start with dry hair in your natural form, whether it's straight, wavy, or curly.

2

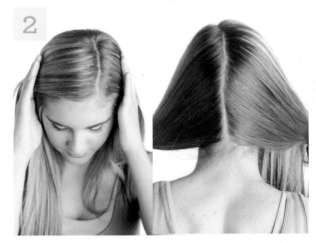

Part out a section of hair with your rattail comb starting at the center of your left eye as a reference point and drawing a line straight back, over, and down the back of your head.

3

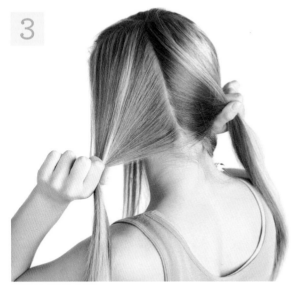

Keeping this section low and at the nape of your neck, separate it into two equal-size subsections. (Feel free to clip any of the sections to separate them or keep them out of the way.)

4

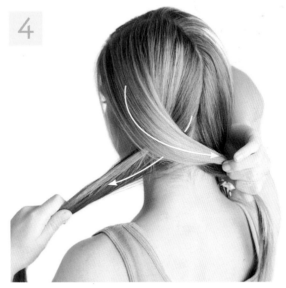

Hold the right subsection down with one hand and using your other hand, twist the left subsection over the right. Now the right is on the left and the left is on the right.

5

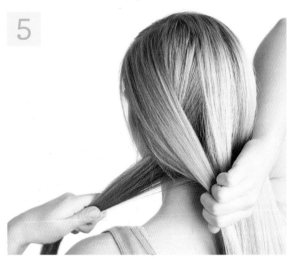

Unclip the hair from the right side, if you clipped it earlier. Grab a vertical section of hair parallel to your first section in step 2, and add that section into the right side of your twist.

6

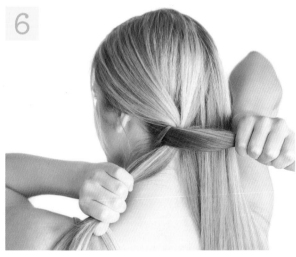

Hold your newly thicker right subsection down toward the nape of your neck as you twist the left side over the right.

7

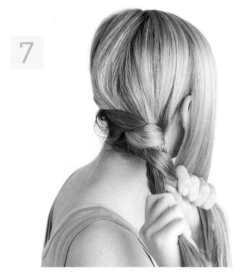

Continue with steps 5 and 6 until your twist reaches the opposite side of your head. When you reach the side, you can add your bangs or the front section of your hair into the ponytail as you twist. Or you can leave out your bangs for a more casual look.

8

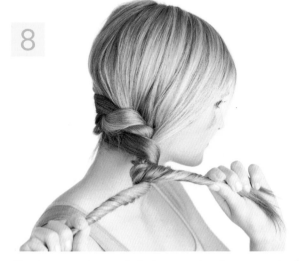

Continue to twist your hair downward to the very ends of your hair. To keep your twisted pony from unraveling, twist each section in opposite directions.

9

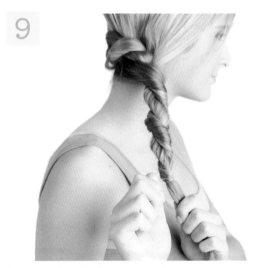

Secure with a clear elastic band.

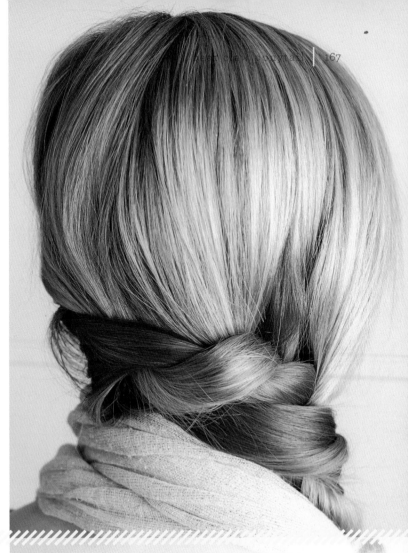

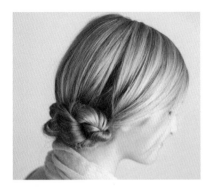

Once you have secured your twist, you can wrap it up in a bun and secure it with hairpins for a fancier look.

For a variation on this pony, stop twisting when you reach the opposite side of your head, secure your twist, and leave the ends of your hair as a loose ponytail hanging down. If you don't already have naturally wavy or curly hair, you can curl your pony with a medium-barrel curling iron. Then wrap a small piece of hair around your ponytail where the clear elastic band is to cover it. Secure the small piece of hair with a bobby pin.

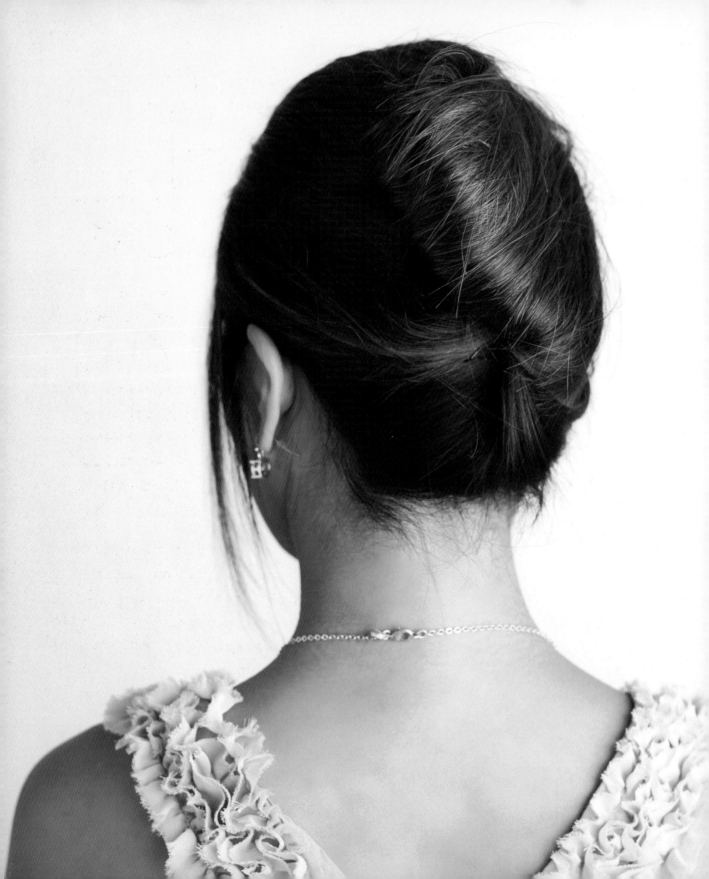

Styles for SPECIAL OCCASIONS

When a special occasion arises, what are your first thoughts? What you'll wear? What shoes you'll don? How you'll style your hair? If this is your line of thinking, you're far from alone. Open a magazine, log on to a website, or turn on your television and you can see wonderful hairstyles gracing the red carpet and award shows. Think you can't possibly re-create those same styles at home? Think again—it's easy!

In this part, I share several classic styles, such as the Simple Chignon and French Twist, as well as offer a new variety of looks, like the Broken Fishbone and Retro Waves. These styles allow you to divulge your inner artist and create your own up-dos and formal styles—all while in the comfort of your own home. Soon, you'll be creating your own polished, professional-looking styles.

Simple Chignon

When you walk into a room wearing this chic bun, you exude elegance. This formal style is a classic low-slung bun of sorts that can be a jumping-off point for a variety of other looks. Try a more casual, modern version during the day worn with a headband for a boho twist. The dressier interpretation can span from a quinceañera to walking down the aisle on your wedding day. The possibilities are endless for all hair textures.

TOOLS NEEDED

bobby pins

clear elastic band

hairpins (optional)

medium- to firm-hold hairspray

rattail comb

teasing comb

PREPPING YOUR HAIR | You can leave your hair in its natural state—straight or curly—to begin this style.

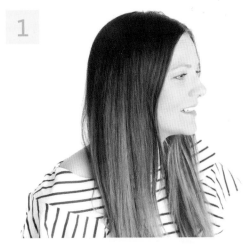

1

Start with dry hair in your natural form, whether it's straight, wavy, or curly.

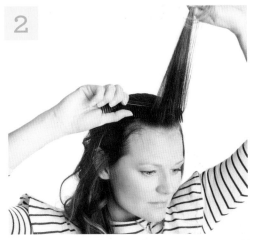

2

Separate a section of hair about 1 inch (2.5cm) from your hairline. Hold this hair up at 90 degrees from your scalp, and use a teasing comb to gently tease your hair.

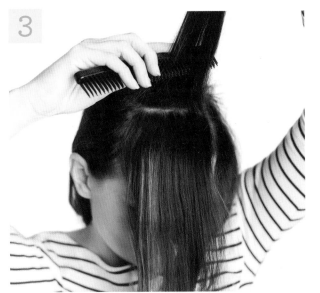

3

Separate a second section in your crown area, directly behind the first, and tease that section, too.

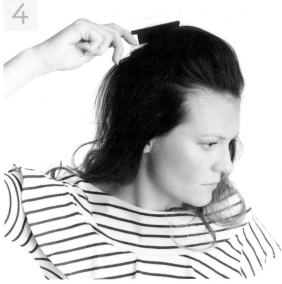

4

Continue teasing the hair in your crown until you have a lot of volume on top. Use a rattail comb to very carefully comb over your teased area to smooth the rough edges.

For additional fullness, you can tease the sides of your hair as well.

5

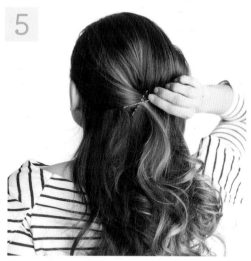

Pick up one side of your hair like you're going to put it half-up style, and swing it to the back of your head. Secure this section with bobby pins, crossing two pins in an X to make your hair more secure.

6

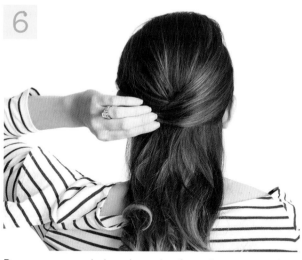

Repeat step 5 with the other side of your hair, pinning this section up and under the first so the pins don't show. You should now have a voluminous half-up hairdo.

7

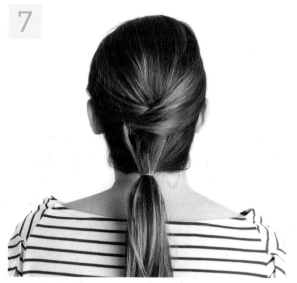

Gather all of your hair, including the bottom of your half-up hairdo, and secure into a loose, low ponytail using a clear elastic band.

8

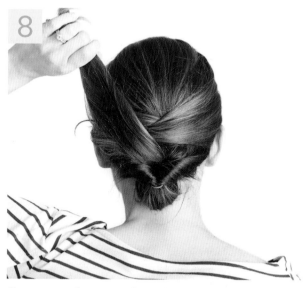

Create a small opening above the elastic band at the base of your ponytail using two of your fingers. Reach down through the opening, grab your ponytail, and pull it through the opening.

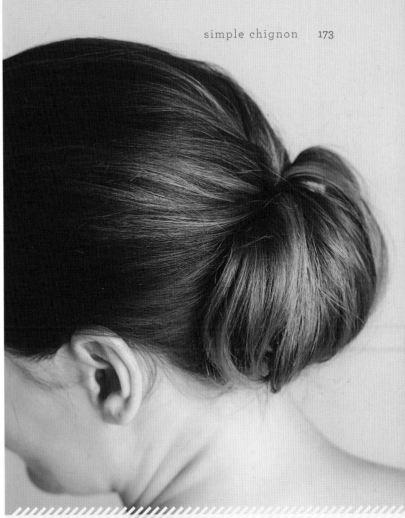

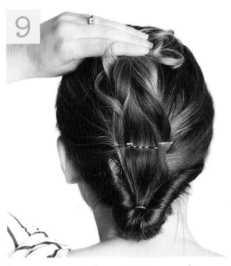

9

Repeat step 8 to invert your ponytail again, and pin it horizontally with bobby pins.

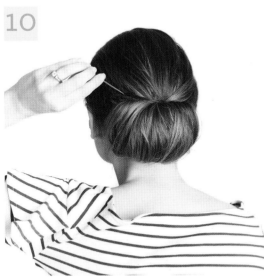

10

Tuck the remaining ends of your ponytail down at the nape of your neck to produce a bun. Secure any loose ends with hairpins and/or bobby pins. Finish with a medium- to firm-hold hairspray to tame unruly hairs and set the style.

For a slightly more casual style, after step 7, place a headband around your head about 1 or 2 inches (2.5 to 5cm) from your hairline—or just behind your bangs if you have them. Be sure to place the headband over and on top of the clear elastic band. Then, when you make the opening for the ponytail to slip through, make it above the band so you can pull your ponytail around the headband as you're inverting your pony.

Retro Waves

This style is reminiscent of the glamorous looks actresses like Bette Davis, Veronica Lake, and Lauren Bacall wore in the 1940s. Dressed-up tresses such as these are meant for special occasions or fashion-forward gatherings. Almost all hair types are suited for these swirls.

TOOLS NEEDED

boar bristle paddle brush

clips

curling iron with a 1-inch (2.5cm) barrel

duckbill clips

medium-hold hairspray

pomade

working hairspray

PREPPING YOUR HAIR | Before blow-drying your hair, prep it with a holding product to help enhance your curls. If you have wavy or curly hair, soften it first with an antihumectant and frizz-resistant serum before applying a light- or strong-hold gel, depending on thickness of your hair. If you have fine hair and need an extra boost, apply a root lifter, followed by an amplifying mousse.

1

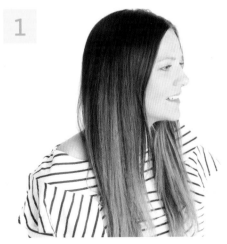

Start with dry hair that's been blown out, or with smooth hair that's been prepped with the proper styling products.

2

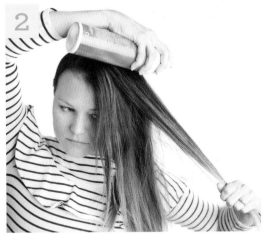

Apply a working hairspray all over your hair to prime it for the curling iron.

3

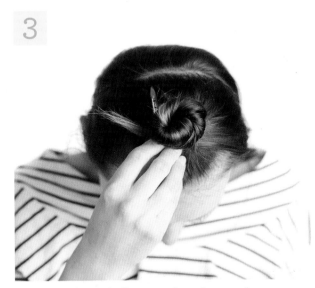

Divide your hair in half, parting from the top of one ear over the top of your head and down to the top of your other ear. Clip all your hair in the top section out of the way.

4

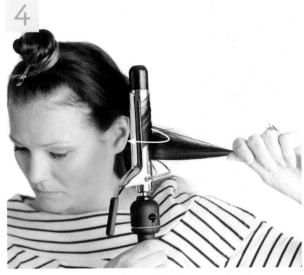

Pull out a subsection of hair about 2 or 3 inches (5 to 7.5cm) wide closest to your face. Using a curling iron with a 1-inch (2.5cm) barrel, curl toward your face.

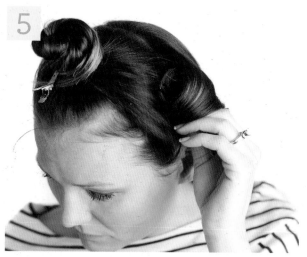

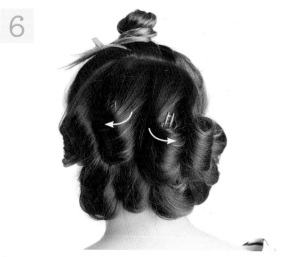

As you finish each curl, drop the curl lightly into your palm, wrap the curl back up around your fingers, place a duckbill clip inside the curl, and clip it to the hair at your scalp to set the curl.

Continue curling around your head in the bottom section, curling your hair toward your face and clipping your curls to your head until the bottom section is curled.

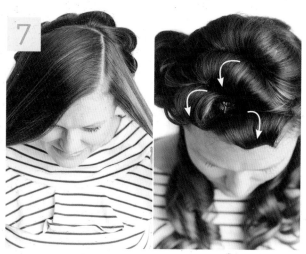

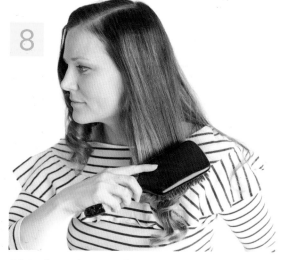

Drop the top section of your hair, and create a deep side part. Curl your hair upward and toward your face, but away from your part for maximum height, until you have the top section all curled.

After all your hair is curled and has had time to set (5 to 10 minutes), release all your curls from the duckbill clips. Brush your hair thoroughly with a boar bristle paddle brush.

9

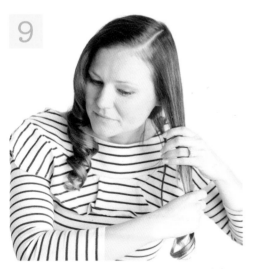

Run pomade over your waves to add polish to your modern retro look, and set your strands with a medium-hold hairspray.

For extra panache, pin the side of your hair opposite your part away from your face and secure it with bobby pins. Add a vintage broach or demure hair accessory to adorn your 'do.

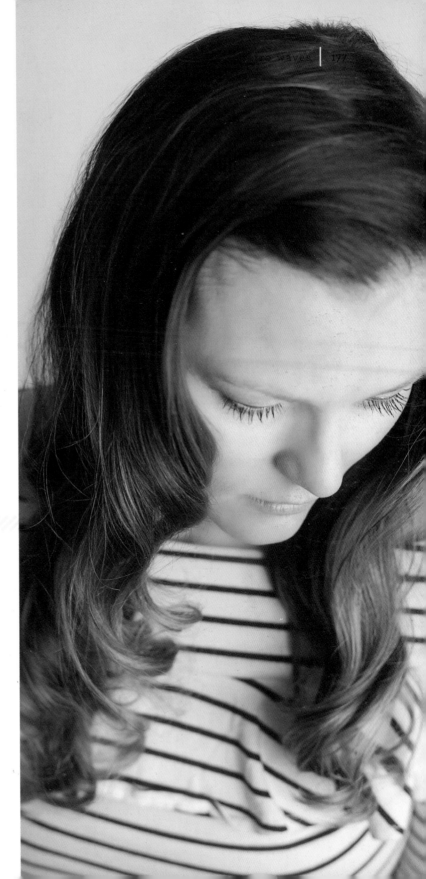

Fishtail Bun

The Fishtail Bun offers an earthy, organic style that's still quite eye-catching. If you're a fan of the messy bun, you'll love this look. It's a simple way to achieve a low-maintenance 'do with high-maintenance appeal. The low-slung bun can be worn out shopping on a Saturday with girlfriends, at a summer concert festival, or even when walking down the aisle. All hair except extremely curly types (it's better to blow curly hair out a bit first) can work this style—in just about 10 minutes!

TOOLS NEEDED

antihumectant hairspray

blow-dryer

bobby pins

clear elastic bands

concentrator

hairpins

paddle brush

teasing comb (optional)

PREPPING YOUR HAIR | Before blow-drying, be sure to use a holding product to help your style last longer. You don't want pieces of your hair to come undone. Use a volumizer on your roots for lift in your crown and either a volumizing foam or sculpting lotion for the middle and ends of your hair.

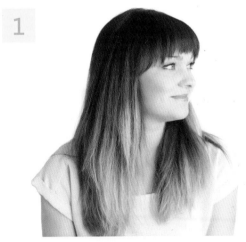

Start with thoroughly towel-dried hair.

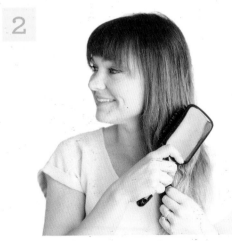

Apply a holding product evenly throughout your hair, and use a paddle brush to further distribute the product by brushing until smooth.

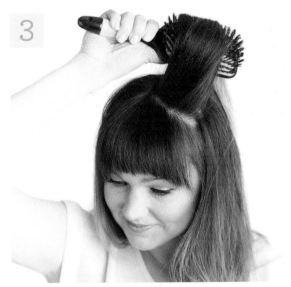

Using the paddle brush, pick up a section of hair at the roots, and slightly turn the brush up and back to create a little bubble in your hair.

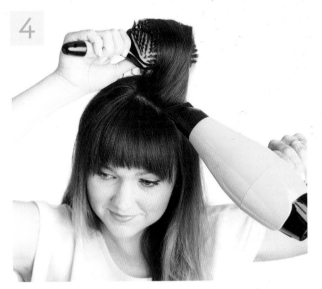

Point the blow-dryer, fitted with a concentrator, close to the roots and upward toward the brush holding the bubbled-over hair. This creates volume without the need to round brush or tease your whole head.

5

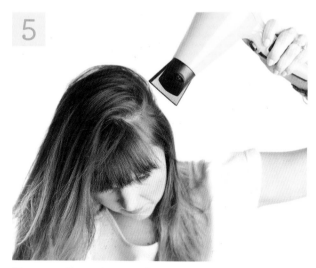

Continue drying the rest of your hair in a back and forth motion until it's dry.

6

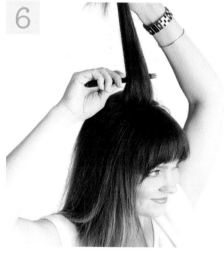

If you want, when your hair is completely dry, you can use a teasing comb to tease your crown area for more volume.

7

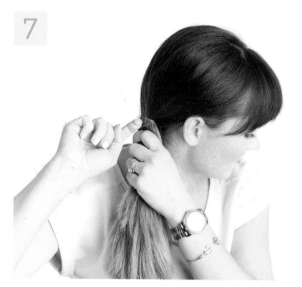

Gather your hair into a low side ponytail, and secure it with a clear elastic band.

8

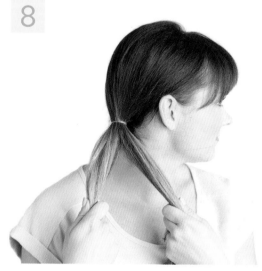

Divide your pony into two equal sections.

9

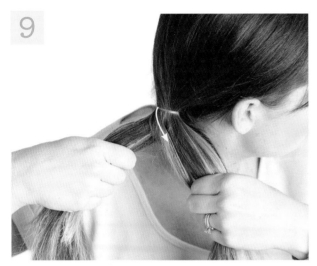

Pick up a piece of hair on the outer right side of the right section, and pull it over and into the left section. That small section is now a part of the left side.

10

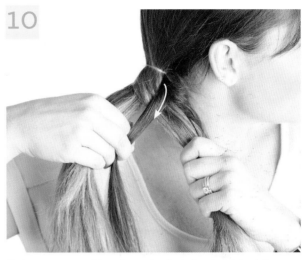

Pick up a piece of hair from the far left side of the left section, and cross it over the top and into the right section. The left piece is now a part of the right section.

11

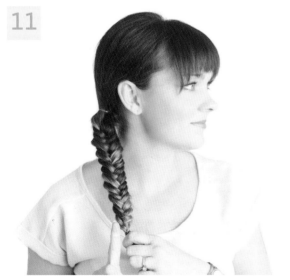

Repeat steps 9 and 10 until your entire ponytail is fishtail braided. Secure the end with a clear elastic band.

12

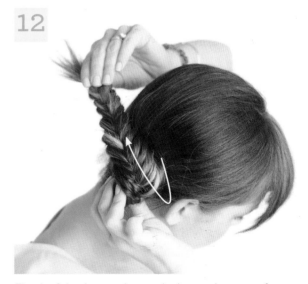

Flip the fishtail upward, onto the hair at the nape of your neck. The fishtail is now inside out or flipped up and to the opposite side.

13

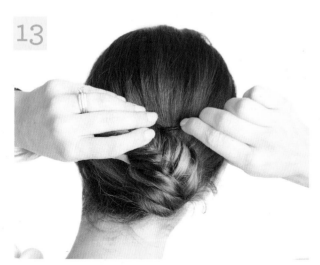

Secure the fishtail with hairpins by pinning the edges (sides) of the tail into the hair at the base of your original ponytail.

14

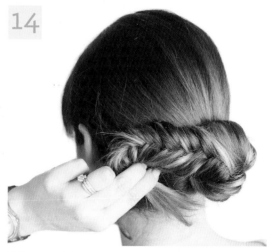

When the fishtail is secure against your head, turn under the ends of your fishtail, and secure it with a bobby pin. Try to hide the clear elastic band if you can.

15

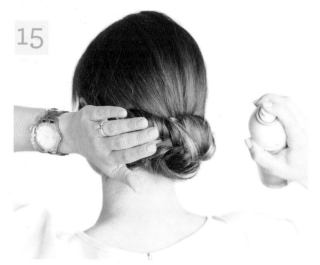

Finish with an antihumectant hairspray.

For an ethereal feel, you can pull apart the fishtail a bit to make it a little loose and slightly messy. Pin any additional unruly hairs with hairpins.

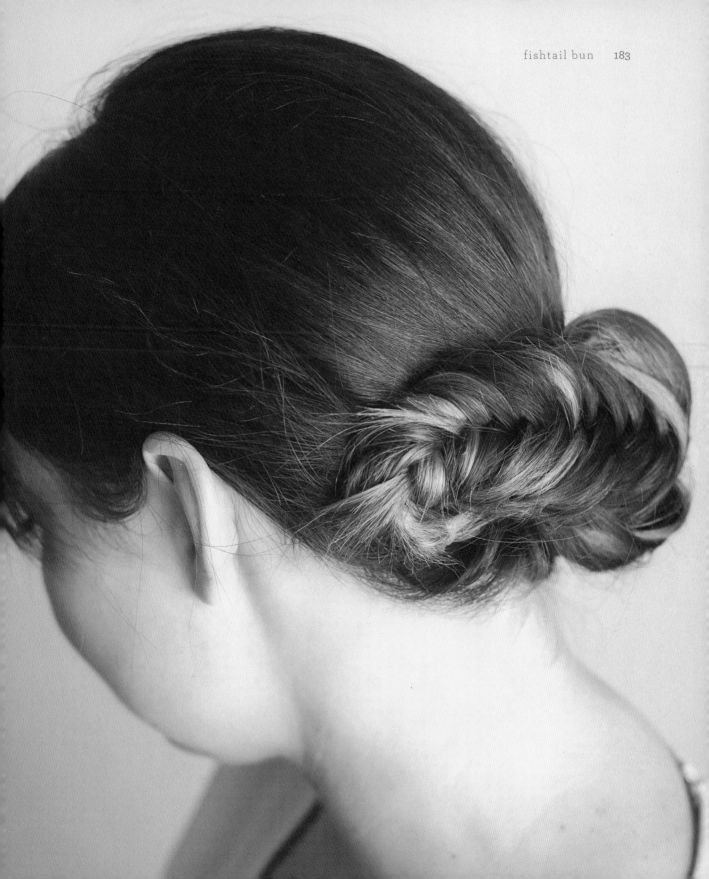

Twisted Pony

The standard ponytail could use a modern update to take you from dinner to date night. This version is an adaptation of the rope braid with a twist—literally! The Twisted Pony works with all textures of hair and can be worn more casually with jeans and a T-shirt on the weekends as well as out for special occasions. Although it's a more formal style, you can make it feel a bit more natural by pulling out some soft hairs around your hairline. Have fun with it!

TOOLS NEEDED

- bobby pin
- clear elastic bands
- clips
- dry shampoo
- medium- to firm-hold hairspray
- teasing comb

PREPPING YOUR HAIR | Let your hair dry naturally if you have wavy or curly hair. If you have straight hair, add some texture with a curling iron or wand before beginning the style.

1

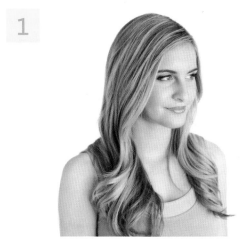

Start with dry hair.

2

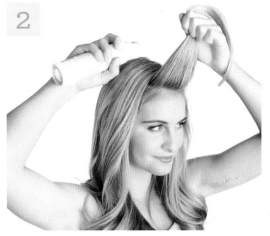

Spray a couple shots of dry shampoo on your roots in your crown area for added volume.

3

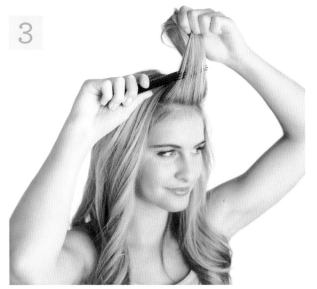

Lift sections of hair in your crown area and tease with a teasing comb. When your entire crown is teased, gently comb over it to create a smooth texture on the top.

4

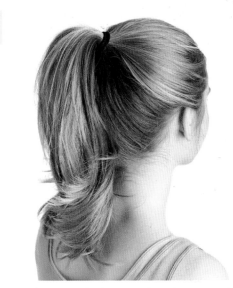

Gather your hair into a high ponytail, and secure with a clear elastic band.

5

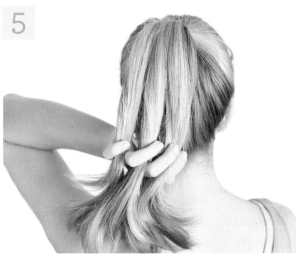

Separate your ponytail into three equal sections.

6

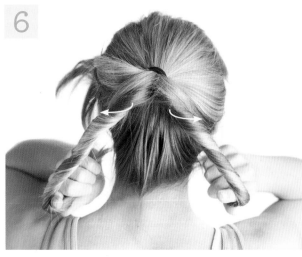

Clip the left section out of the way, being careful not to mess up the smoothness of your pulled-back hair, and twist the remaining two sections separately but simultaneously outward.

7

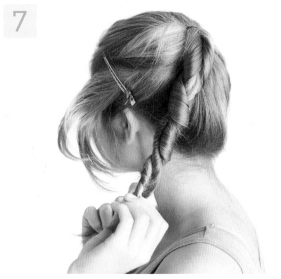

When you've twisted the two sections to the ends, twist the two sections around each other.

8

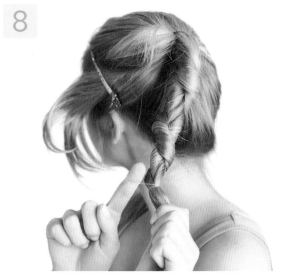

Secure the end of your twists with a clear elastic band.

9

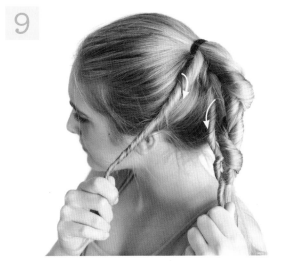

Unclip the section of hair from the left side, divide it into two equal subsections, and twist both sections inward until you reach the ends.

10

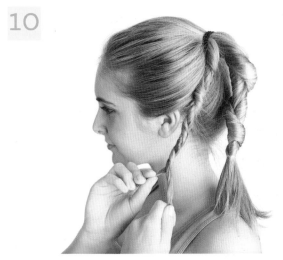

Wrap those two pieces around each other until you've reached the ends. Secure with a clear elastic band if you need to.

11

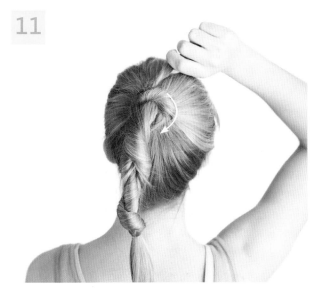

Wrap the rope braid you created with steps 9 and 10 around the base of the ponytail you created in the very beginning.

12

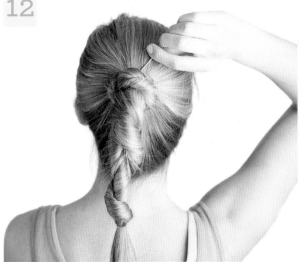

After the rope braid is wound completely around the original ponytail base, secure it with a bobby pin.

13

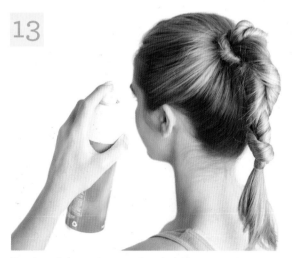

Finish with a medium- to firm-hold hairspray for hold and to tame any unruly hairs.

If you prefer a more natural look, you can pull out small pieces of hair around your hairline before step 13.

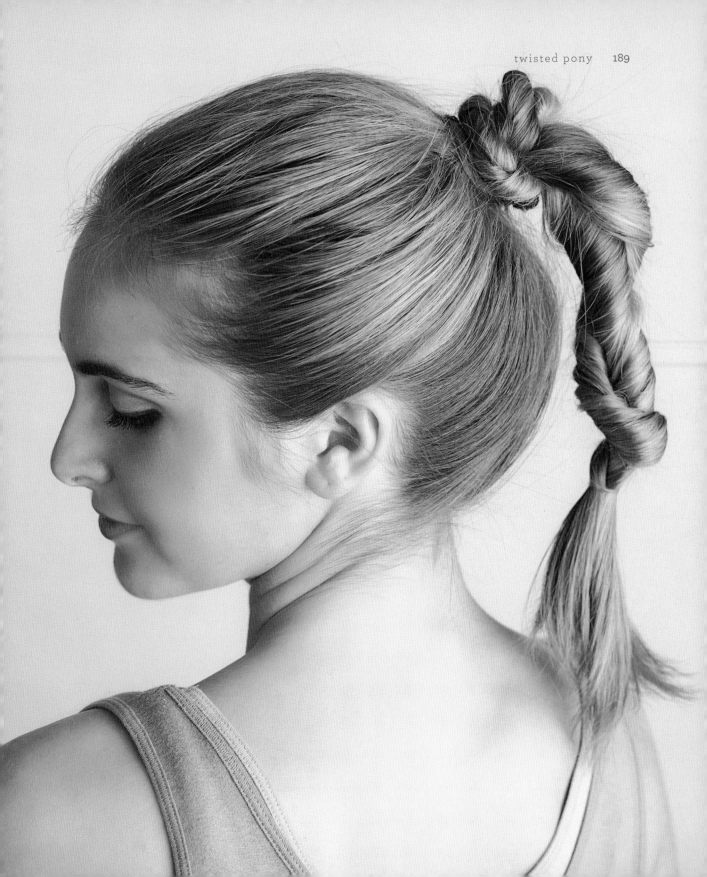

French Twist

The French Twist was at the height of fashion in the 1960s and has continued to be a classic style ever since. This up-do is très chic *and is often worn at proms, weddings, and even formal office settings. More recently, the French Twist has transformed into a more casual style with a loose and airy feel, perfect for those with more natural texture in their hair.*

TOOLS NEEDED

clips (optional)
hairpins
hairspray
paddle brush
teasing comb

PREPPING YOUR HAIR | You want your hair to be relatively smooth to start this style. If you have curly or wavy locks, blow them out first. If you have straight hair, this step might not be necessary for you, but you're free to blow it out first for extra smoothness.

1

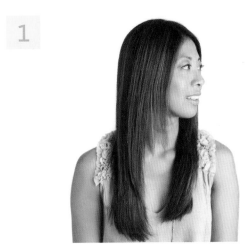

Start with dry hair.

2

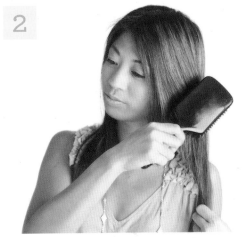

Using a paddle brush, thoroughly brush through your hair to remove any tangles or snags and promote smoothness.

3

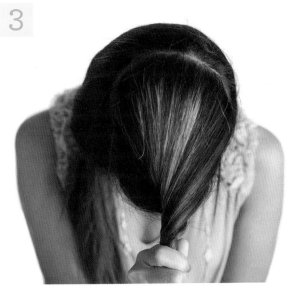

Part out a small section of hair from the recession point on one side of your head to the other in a U shape. You can clip the bottom section out of the way if you like.

4

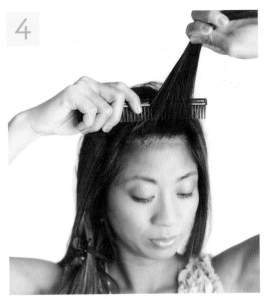

Using a teasing comb, tease this entire section to create soft, subtle volume.

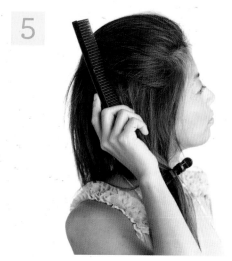

After you've teased this section, very gently comb the outer layer to smooth it.

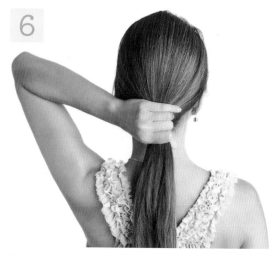

Gather your hair into a low ponytail with your hands.

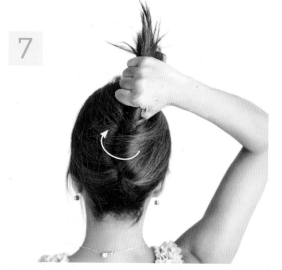

Using your right hand, twist your ponytail clockwise, moving your hand slightly upward until your twist is upside down with the ends of your hair reaching up past your crown.

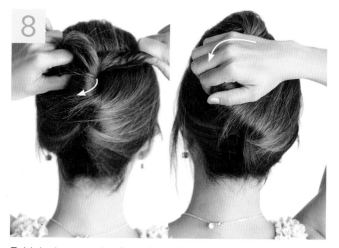

Fold the loose ends of your hair downward and tuck them into the twist. You can use a finger on your left hand to help fold over your twisted section.

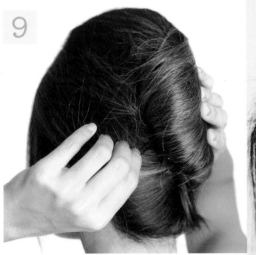

9

After you've tucked as much as possible into the twist, secure all the loose ends with hairpins.

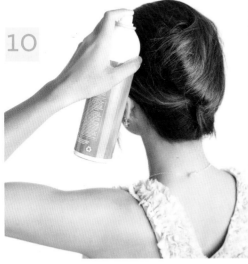

10

Finish with a light veil of hairspray.

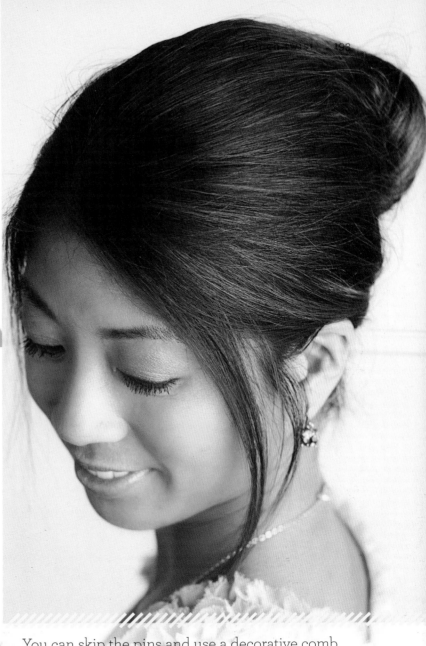

You can skip the pins and use a decorative comb instead. Many brides have used this accessory to add a little sparkle to their wedding-day style. If you opt for this look, spray your comb with hairspray first, and tame any flyaways with an antihumectant pomade. You can use some shine spray to give your hair extra illumination, too.

Side-Swept Pony

The Side-Swept Pony, a special-occasion style without pretention, is hugely popular among teens headed to the prom, brides-maids, and even brides. Thanks to American music stars like Carrie Underwood and Taylor Swift, this pony doesn't seem to be going out of style any-time soon. All hair types can attempt this look.

TOOLS NEEDED

bobby pins

clear elastic band

clips

curling iron with a
1-inch (2.5cm) or
1¼-inch (3cm) barrel

duckbill clips

hairpins (optional)

teasing comb

PREPPING YOUR HAIR | For this look, you want plenty of natural volume. You can blow out your hair if you have wavy or curly locks, but be sure to still have some volume in it.

1

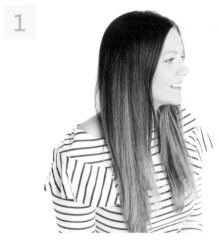

Start with dry hair.

2

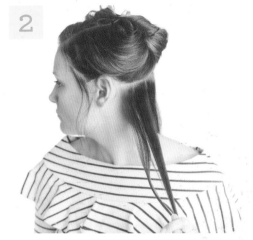

Using a 1- or 1¼-inch (2.5 or 3cm) curling iron, and working with 2-inch (5cm) sections for more efficient curls, curl your hair away from your face.

3

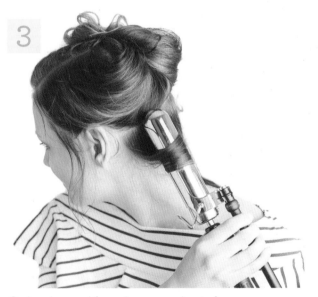

Curl each strand from the root to the tip for a more voluminous look.

4

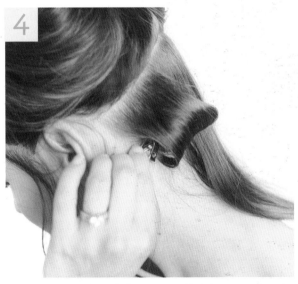

As you finish each curl, drop the curl lightly into your palm, wrap the curl back up around your fingers, place a duckbill clip inside the curl, and clip it to the hair at your scalp to set the curl.

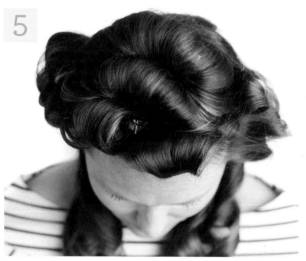

Continue curling and pinning until your entire head is full of pinned curls. After your curls have cooled completely (5 to 10 minutes), remove the clips.

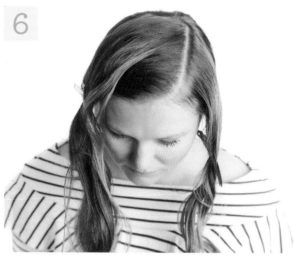

Separate your hair into two sections by parting from the top of one ear to the top of your other ear. Clip all the hair in the front along your hairline out of the way.

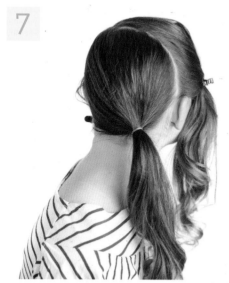

Gather the back section of your hair into a low side ponytail so it rests on your shoulder, and secure it with a clear elastic band.

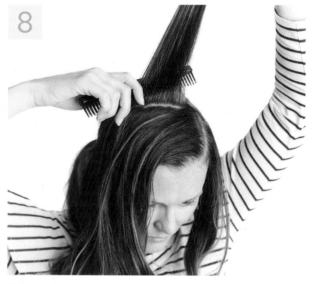

Release the front section. Using a teasing comb, tease your crown and then gently comb over it to smooth out any unruly bits.

9

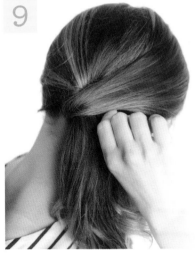

Start to swing that top section toward your low side ponytail. Using bobby pins or hairpins, pin to secure the top section to the bottom.

10

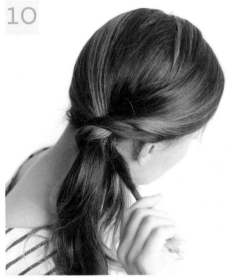

You should still have one small subsection left in front of your ear on the side of the ponytail. Either twist this section in front of your ponytail to hide the elastic band, or wrap it around the elastic band. Secure it with a bobby pin, leaving the ends down to mingle with your ponytail.

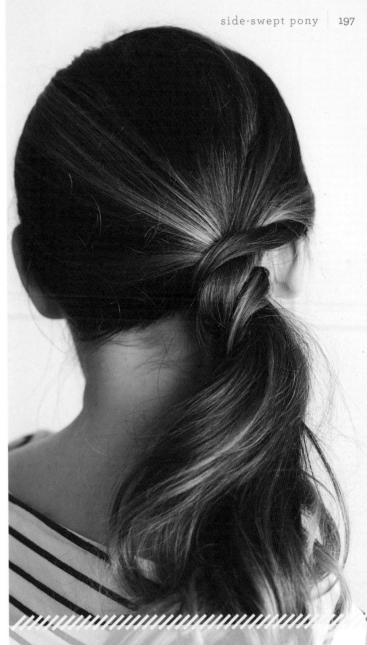

Depending on the length of your bangs or your layers at your front hairline, you can to drop a few pieces of hair to soften the look. And for extra sparkle, adorn your pony with a decorative barrette or broach.

Broken Fishbone

This modern up-do will earn you lots of attention—your friends will beg you to tell them how you created it! The Broken Fishbone is a chignon that appears to be especially intricate but is actually quite simple. Brides will be radiant in this style as will those who are looking for a fresh new twist on evening-out hair. All hair textures work with this look.

TOOLS NEEDED

bobby pins
clear elastic bands
hairpins (optional)
rattail comb

PREPPING YOUR HAIR | Before starting this style, use a curling iron with a 2-inch (5 cm) barrel to add texture to your hair if it's naturally straight.

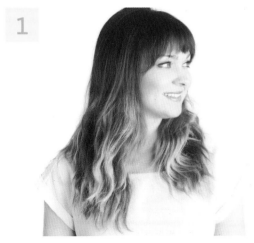

Start with dry hair.

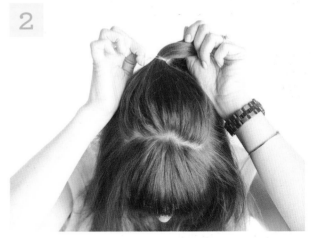

Using a rattail comb, gather a U-shape section of hair from the recession point on one side of your hairline to the recession point on the other side. Secure this section of hair at the back of your head with a clear elastic band.

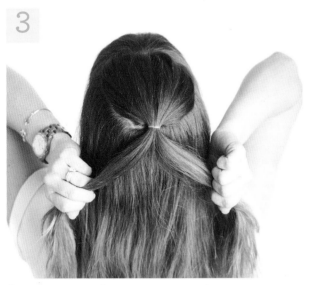

Separate your small pony into two equal sections.

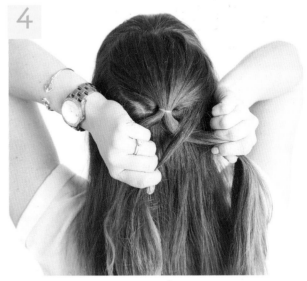

Pick up a horizontal section of hair directly beneath the front part of your ponytail on the right side. Cross this section of hair over and add it to the left section your left hand is holding.

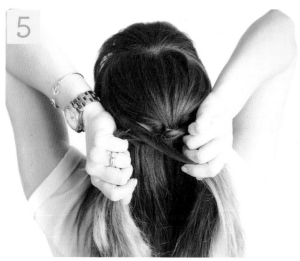

Pick up a horizontal section beneath the pony area on the left side. Cross it over and add it to the right section. Your right hand remains on the right section.

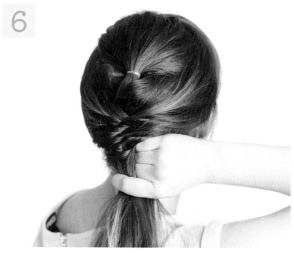

Repeat steps 4 and 5 until you reach the nape of your neck.

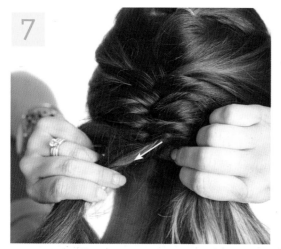

When you reach your nape, begin to braid the rest of your hair in a classic fishtail, grabbing a small outer piece of hair from the right side and crossing it over and into the left section.

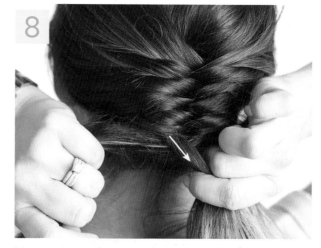

Next, grab a small outer section of hair from the left side and cross it over and into the right side. This whole time, your right hand remains on the right section of your hair and your left hand on the left section.

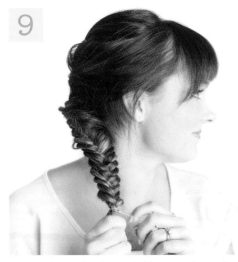

Secure the ends of your fishbone with another clear elastic band.

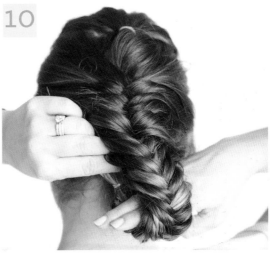

Wrap the end of the fishbone tail around your index and middle fingers to coil it upward.

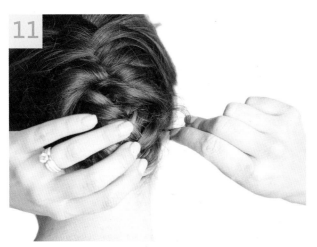

Curl the coil up to the French-braided fishtail, tuck it up and underneath it, and secure it with bobby pins. You also can add hairpins for any layers or stray hairs that have fallen out of place during the styling process.

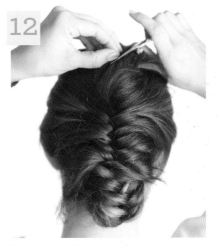

If your fishtail is low and doesn't cover the clear elastic band, you can cut and remove the band.

For added glamour and urban hippie appeal, add a headscarf or headband.

Half Twist

Based on the classic French twist, this modern, twisted up-do gives your hair a new persona. Instead of twisting upward, this adaptation twists the hair downward using three smaller twists instead of one. It can look very stylish with bangs or just as fab without. If you prefer a loose, easy vibe with your hair, this style will be a great fit for you because it's very versatile and never appears rigid or stiff. Wear it to an art gala or even to a local summer street fair. All textures can achieve this twist, but it'll be easier to create if your hair is at least to your shoulders.

TOOLS NEEDED

bobby pins
clear elastic band
clips
curling iron with a
1-inch (2.5cm) barrel

medium-hold
hairspray
paddle brush
teasing comb

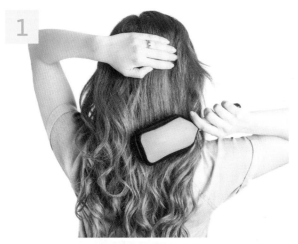

Start with dry hair. Thoroughly brush through your hair with a paddle brush to remove any tangles.

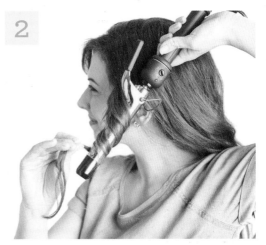

Working with a small, vertical subsection of hair next to your hairline, and using a 1-inch (2.5cm) curling iron with the tip pointed downward, wrap your hair around the iron, directing your hair away from your face. Once you've wrapped the hair completely around the iron, hold it for about 8 to 10 seconds.

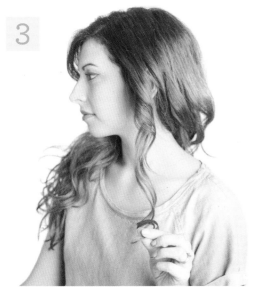

Let the curl drop down from the curling iron, and allow it to cool. Don't rake through it with your fingers.

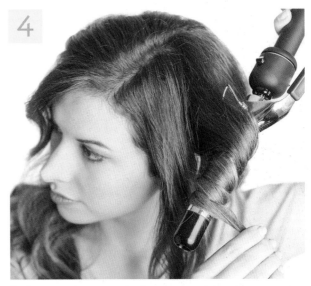

Pick up another vertical subsection at about the same size as the first, and repeat steps 2 and 3 to curl.

5

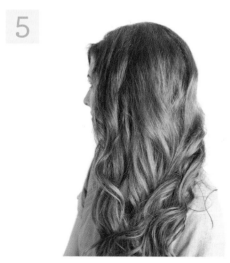

Continue curling until your entire head of hair is curled.

6

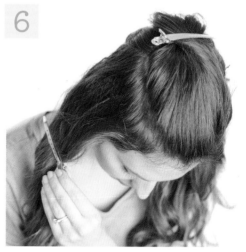

Separate your hair into three sections. First, part your hair starting at the recession point on one side of your head and drawing a line straight back over your head and down. Clip this section out of your way. Next, draw a line straight back and down from your other recession point, and clip that section out of the way.

7

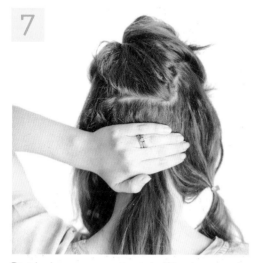

Divide the center section in half by drawing a horizontal line across the top of where your occipital bone is.

Your occipital bone is that knob-feeling bone at the back of your head.

8

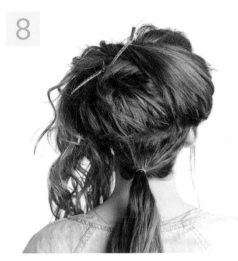

Gather the entire bottom half of your section into a low ponytail, and secure it with a clear elastic band.

9

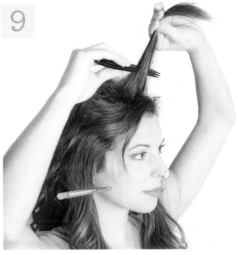

Using a teasing comb, tease the upper half of your center section to create plenty of volume in your crown area.

10

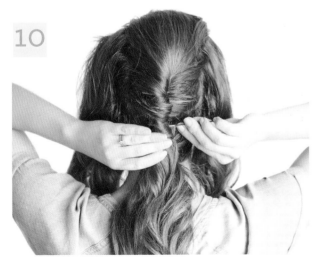

After you've teased your crown, twist it in a downward motion, and pin it in place using bobby pins.

11

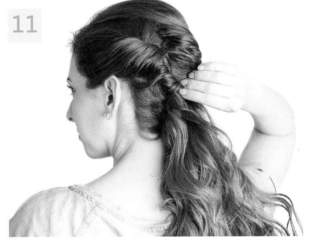

Drop the two outer sections, and gently tease them from the inside. Twist the left section inward and downward toward your first twist. Secure it with bobby pins adjacent to the first twist.

12

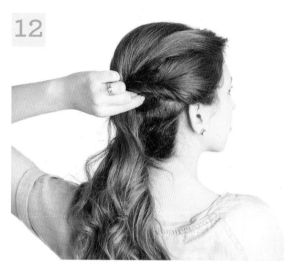

Twist the right side, your final section, inward and downward toward your first twist as well. Pin it with bobby pins to make it secure.

13

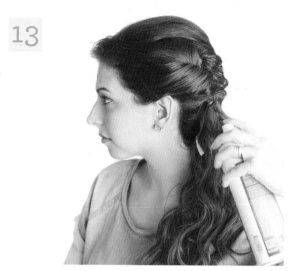

Finish with a spritz of medium-hold hairspray.

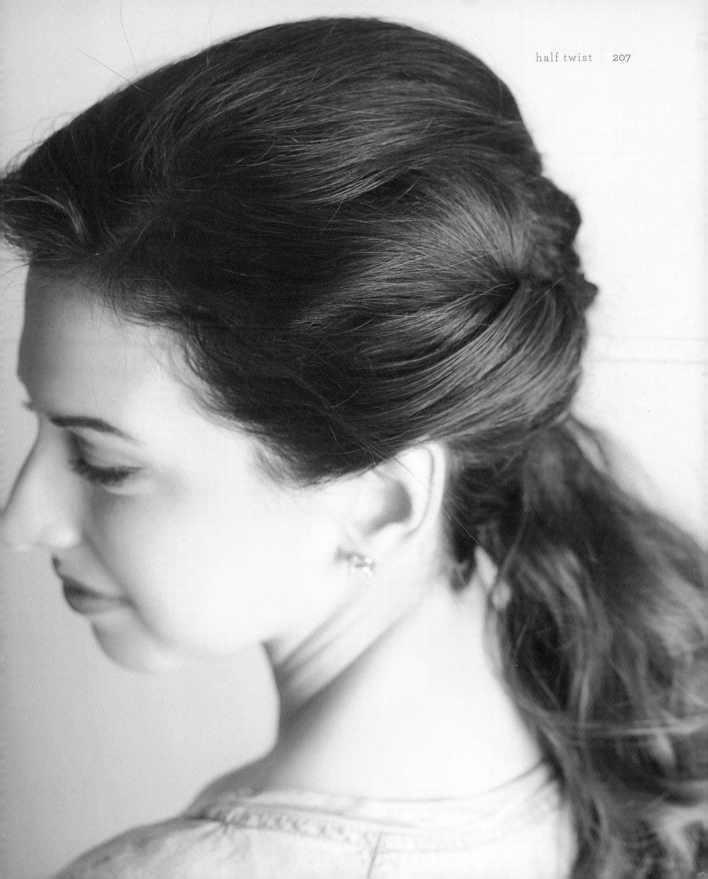

Faux Bob

Love your longer hair but sometimes yearn for a short-hair look? This style allows you to have short hair temporarily, without actually cutting your locks. The Faux Bob has a vintage glam allure that pairs well with special events and has been seen many times on the red carpet and at awards shows. It's a look best suited for dressier occasions, but it could transform into a more casual style with a couple tweaks.

TOOLS NEEDED

boar bristle brush
bobby pins
clear elastic bands
clips
curling iron with a
1-inch (2.5cm) barrel

duckbill clips
firm-hold hairspray
hairpins (optional)
teasing comb

1

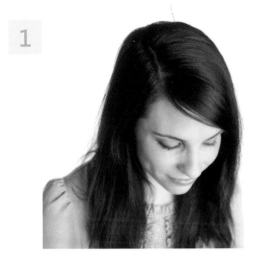

Start with dry hair with a side part.

2

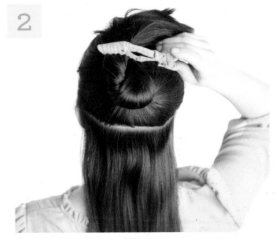

Part your hair horizontally from the top of one ear, around the back of your head, to the top of your other ear. Clip your top section of hair up and out of the way.

3

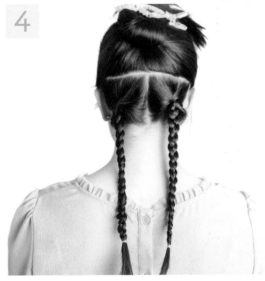

Divide the bottom section into two equal sections.

4

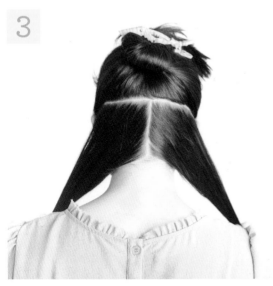

Braid both sections, and secure the ends of the braids with clear elastic bands.

5

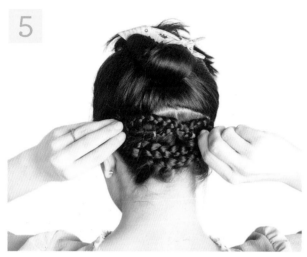

Fold the braids up onto the bottom of the back of your head so they lay as flat as possible. You want them up out of the way against your scalp so they're hidden underneath your top section of hair later. Secure your braids with bobby pins.

6

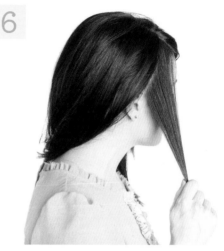

Drop your top section, and divide it into small vertical subsections to prepare for curling.

7

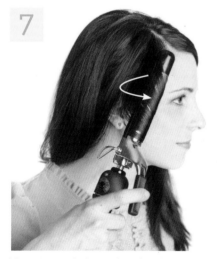

Using a 1-inch (2.5cm) curling iron, curl each subsection forward, toward your face.

8

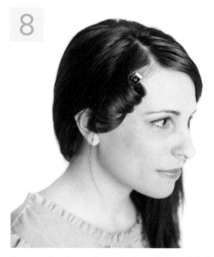

As you finish each curl, drop the curl lightly into your palm, wrap the curl back up around your fingers, place a duckbill clip inside the curl, and clip it to the hair at your scalp to set the curl.

9

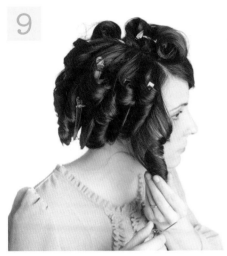

After your entire head has been curled and set with the duckbill clips, remove each clip very carefully so you don't disrupt the curl.

10

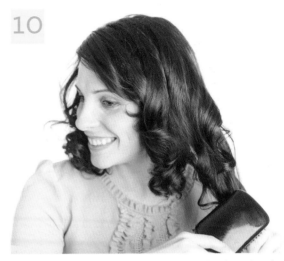

Thoroughly brush through your hair with a boar bristle brush to soften your curls.

11

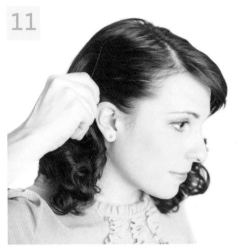

Use a bobby pin to pin one side of your hair back by your ear on the side of your part.

12

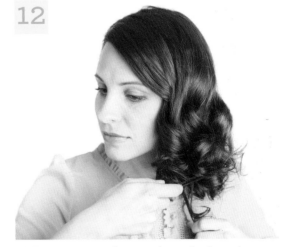

With a teasing comb, tease the ends of your hair to give them added fullness.

13

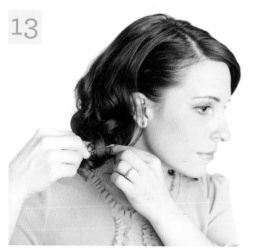

Begin pinning the ends of your hair by tucking the tips up and under and securing with bobby pins or hairpins. Pin just above the ends of your hair so the ends can hang down and make your bob look more realistic. The pins will have plenty to grip onto as you pin into your braids hidden underneath your bob.

14

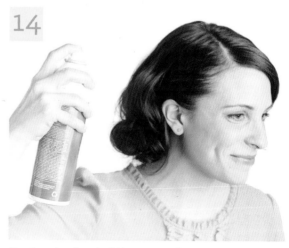

Finish with a firm-hold hairspray. If you plan on dancing, you don't want this style to go anywhere!

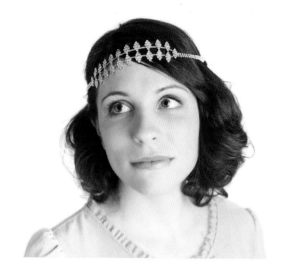

After all your hair has been pinned up, you can slip a headband over the top of your hair for the vintage flapper look.

For a less-formal style, refrain from using the headband and pull out a couple pieces of hair at your hairline. This creates an easy, soft, slightly undone look.

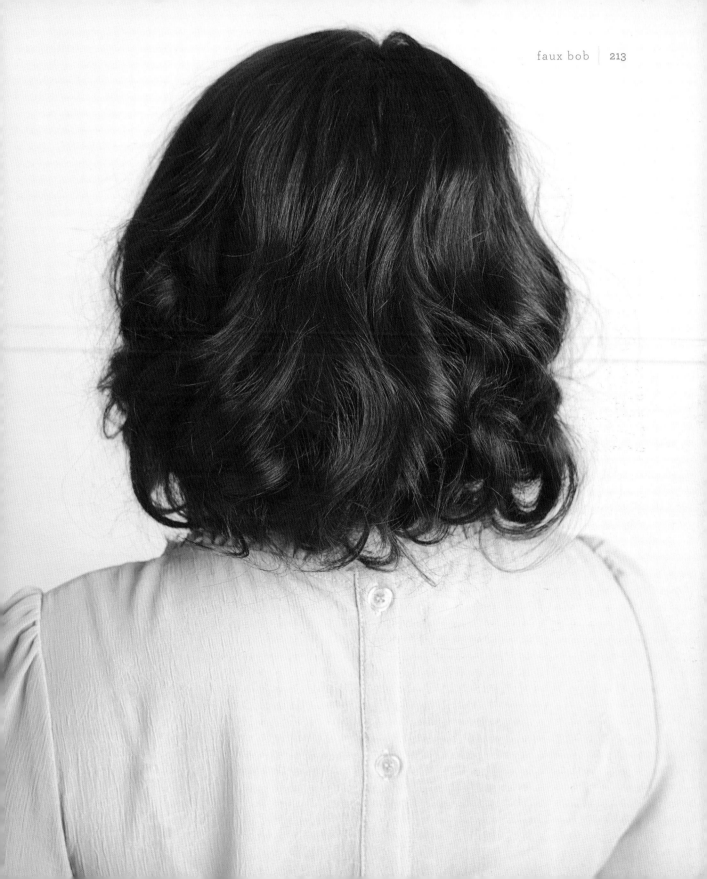

Waterfall Braid

This cascading braid gets its name from the tendrils of hair that fall with perfection down the lengths of your locks. This style is a real crowd pleaser and is sure to earn you countless compliments at your daughter's dance recital, a best friend's wedding, or your city's charity ball. All textures of hair can do this design.

TOOLS NEEDED

antifrizz cream
(optional)
bobby pins
clear elastic band
hairspray (optional)

PREPPING YOUR HAIR | This style
looks the most polished when soft curls are involved. If you
have straight or slightly wavy hair and want to add curl, grab
a curling iron with a 2-inch (5cm) barrel, and curl your hair
starting at your ears and continuing downward.

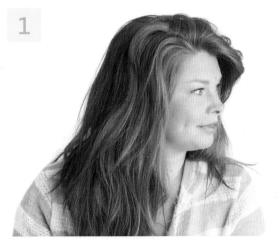

Start with freshly washed and dried hair in its natural state.

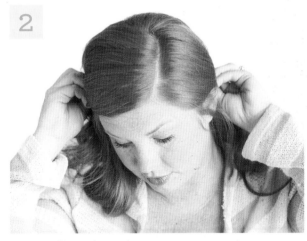

Part your hair either in the center or to one side.

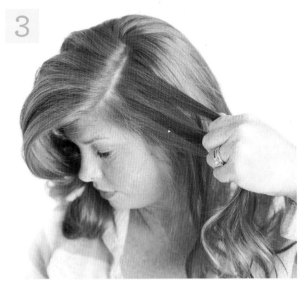

Gather a small section of hair on one side of your head, close to your hairline. Divide this section into three smaller subsections.

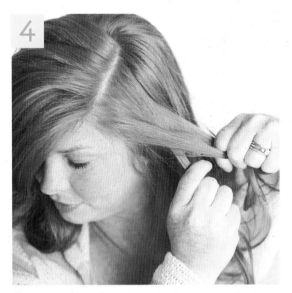

Cross the right subsection over the center subsection. Cross the left subsection over the center subsection as well.

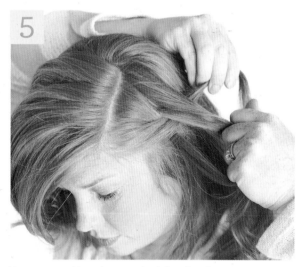

If you started braiding on the left side of your head, grab a small horizontal section from the right side to feed into your braid. Combine the right subsection you have from step 4 and the new section. Hold onto these pieces with your right hand, and fold this section over the center section. (If you started on the right side, grab a section from your left side here.)

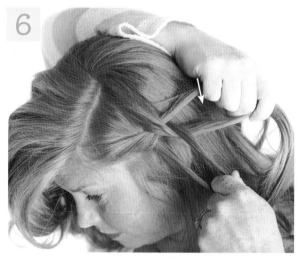

Drop the left section you're holding in your left hand, grab a piece of hair directly behind the section you just dropped, and fold it over the center section.

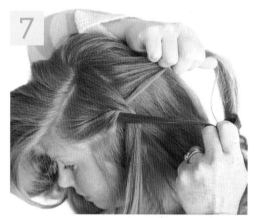

Grab another horizontal section of hair from above the braid. Add this piece to the right section you're already holding on to. Cross this combined section over the center section. Then drop the right side and grab another piece of hair at about the same thickness as the piece you dropped. Cross that piece over the center section. You're always grabbing from the top, above the braid. That's what makes it look like a waterfall.

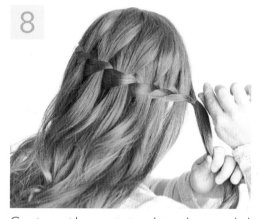

Continue with steps 5, 6, and 7 until you reach the opposite side of your head, just behind your ear. Grab the last section of hair next to your hairline, and pull it backward toward your ear. Secure your finished waterfall braid with bobby pins or a clear elastic band.

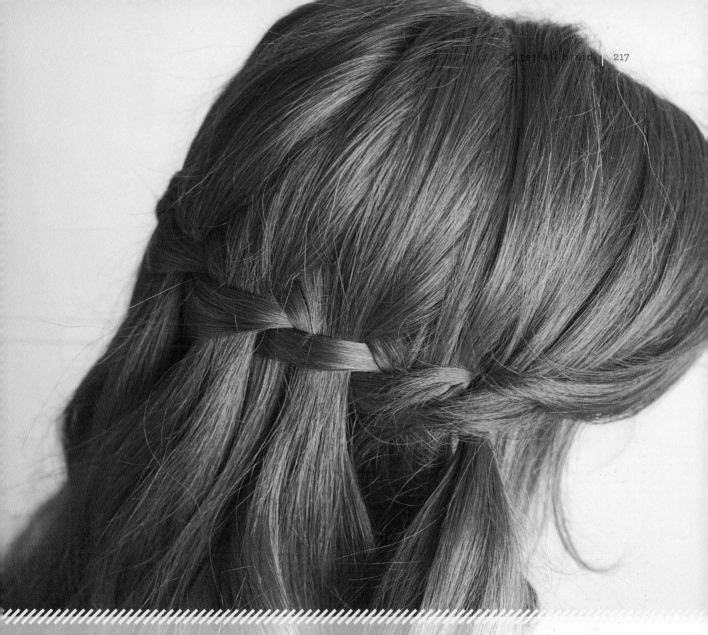

If you have thick hair, you can wrap the ends of your bangs around the ponytail near your ear and secure it with a bobby pin.

You may need to add bobby pins to the sections of hair that are actually doing the "waterfall" because they aren't secured to anything.

If your hair is unruly and in need of some polish, use some antifrizz cream to tame your mane. You also can finish with hairspray for additional hold if needed.

Side Bun

A variation of the classic bun, the Side Bun is sure to quickly become essential in your hairstyle repertoire. This look works well for weddings, proms, and galas. It's best worn to fancy gatherings where you want a refined, elegant style. All hair works with this look that appears to be more time-consuming than it really is.

TOOLS NEEDED

bobby pins

clear elastic band

clips

curling iron with a $1^{1}/_{4}$- to 2-inch (3 to 5cm) barrel (depending on the length of your hair)

hairpins (optional)

long, flat silver clips

medium- to firm-hold hairspray

teasing comb

PREPPING YOUR HAIR | You don't need a lot of prepwork for this style. If you have extremely curly hair, however, you might want to blow it out to loosen your curls. For whatever texture hair you have, you want to eliminate as much frizz as possible.

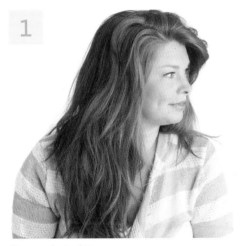

Start with dry hair.

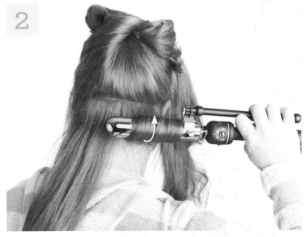

Part your hair horizontally from the top of one ear, behind your head, to the top of your other ear; clip all the top section out of the way; separate your hair into small subsections; and use a 1¹/₄- to 2-inch (3 to 5cm) curling iron to curl your hair upward.

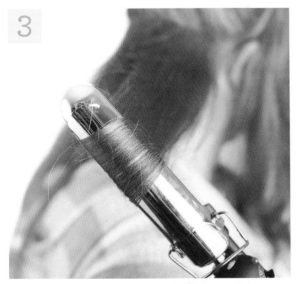

Be sure to include the very tips of your strand in the curl. This ensures the curl is as smooth as possible.

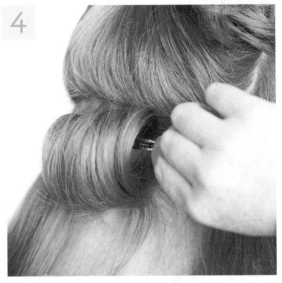

Release the curl from the barrel of your curling iron, roll it back up into the curled position, and secure it to your head with a long, flat silver clip.

5

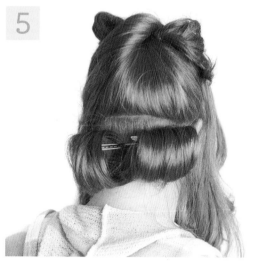

Be sure to use flat clips rather than duckbill clips. The former allow your hair to set without leaving any creases like the latter.

Repeat steps 2, 3, and 4 until the bottom section of your hair is all curled and clipped. After all your curls are set and cool (5 to 10 minutes), remove the clips.

6

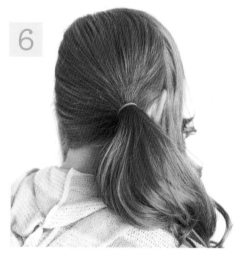

Gather your hair into a low side ponytail, and secure it with a clear elastic band.

7

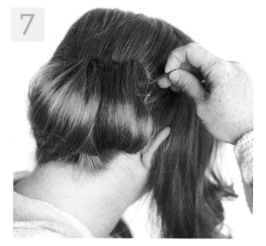

Your hair should naturally want to curl upward in the ponytail because you precurled that area. Roll your ponytail upward, and secure it with bobby pins to the base of your scalp.

8

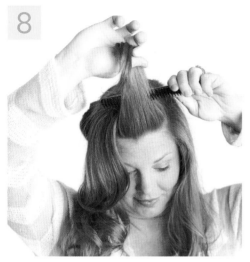

Drop your top section of hair, and use a teasing comb to tease your crown at the roots to create plenty of volume.

9

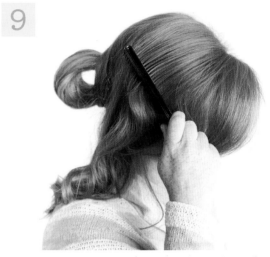

Gently brush over your teased crown to remove any rough patches. This style is meant to stay smooth.

10

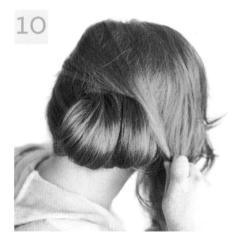

Wrap the ends of your top section around the low bun, and pin any loose hair up and underneath the bun with hairpins or bobby pins.

11

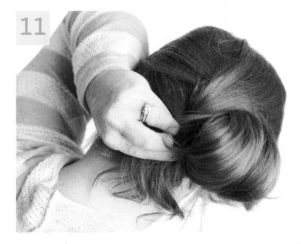

Direct the left side of the bun over to the right side.

12

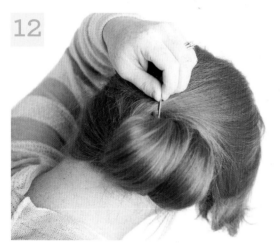

Pin this piece in place with bobby pins or hairpins.

If you prefer to add softness to this style, you can pull out a your bangs or a few short (not long) front pieces. This makes the look more relaxed.

13

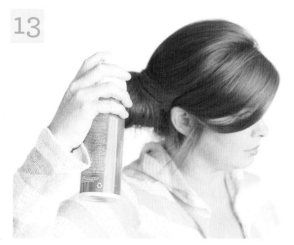

Finish with a medium- to firm-hold hairspray.

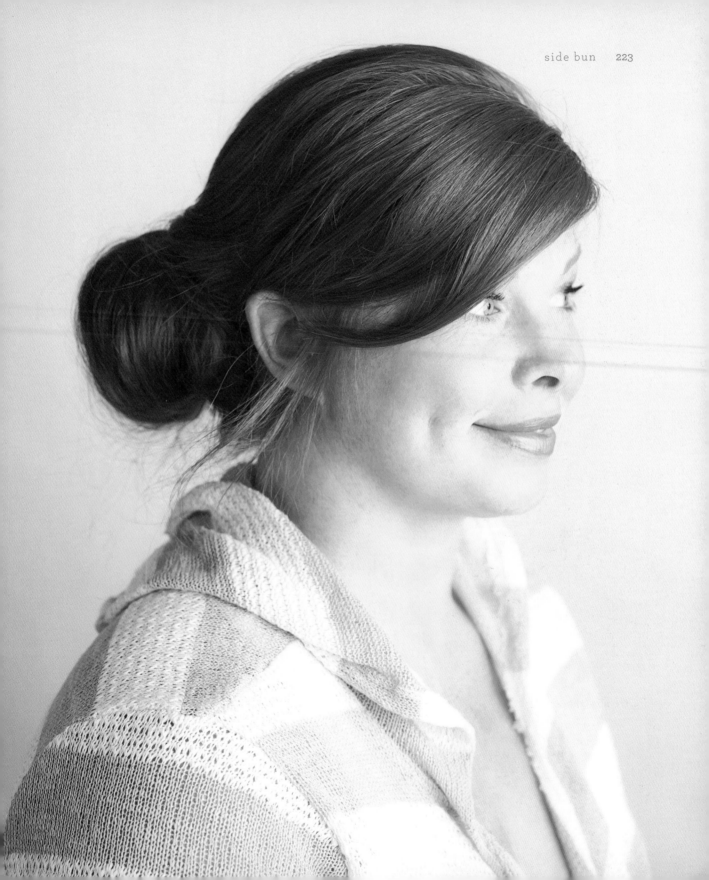

Half Up

Brides around the world are opting for a simpler style for their big day. The Half Up gives a laid-back feel to the typical up-dos commonly worn at weddings. More recently, it's been paired with wreaths of flowers for an organic halo effect. Although it's more relaxed than an up-do style, it still has plenty of polish to be perfect for your special event. All textures and types can achieve this look.

TOOLS NEEDED

bobby pins

curling iron with a 1- to 1¼-inch (2.5- to 3cm) barrel

light-hold hairspray (optional)

spray wax (optional)

teasing comb

PREPPING YOUR HAIR | For a little more volume and grip at your crown, apply a root-lifting foam. If desired, apply it directly to your scalp and rub it into your hair with your fingertips.

1

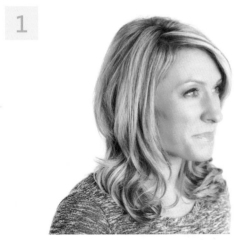

Start with hair that's been dried naturally for added movement.

2

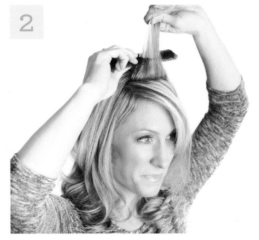

Starting at about 2 inches (5cm) away from your hairline, hold a section of hair at 90 degrees to your scalp, and use a teasing comb to tease your crown. Continue teasing until your entire crown is full of volume.

3

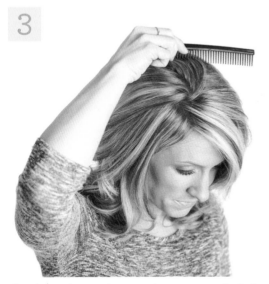

Gently comb over the teased area so you don't disrupt all volume you just created.

4

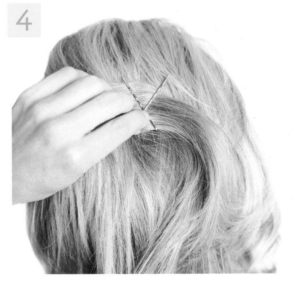

Grab a small section of hair just above your left ear, and pin it across the back of your head with bobby pins. Use the X method of pinning to secure your hair.

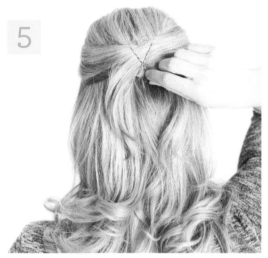

Grab a small section of hair above your right ear, and pull it across the back of your head, past and over the section you just pinned. Pin this section with the X method also.

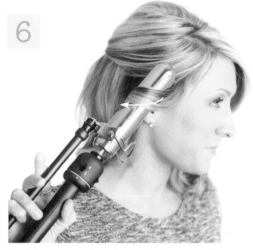

Curl the remainder of your hair hanging downward. It's easiest to grab small vertical subsections and curl away from your face using a curling iron with a 1- to 1¼-inch (2.5- to 3cm) barrel.

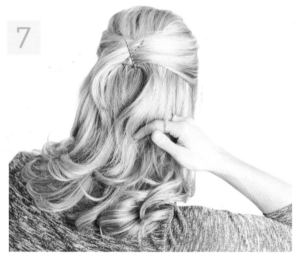

Using your fingers, gently comb through your curls.

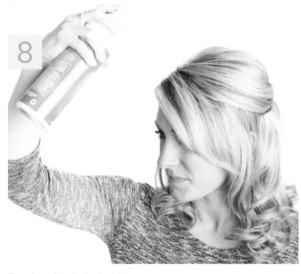

Finish with a light-hold hairspray or a spray wax for additional texture.

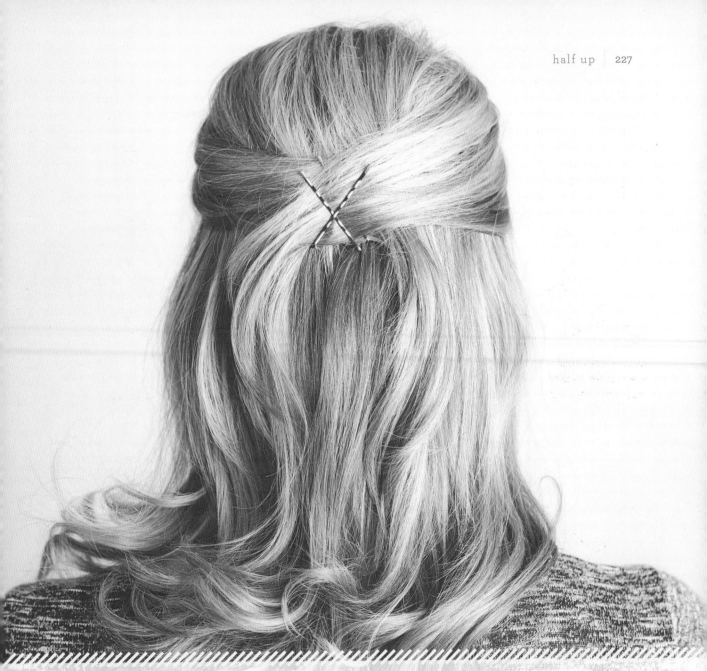

Use a 1-inch (2.5cm) curling iron for a smaller and more uniform curls, and use the 1¼-inch (3cm) iron for a looser, more laid-back look.

You can pin your hair in different ways. For example, you can grab additional pieces from each side of your head, near your ears, to make a basket-weave effect. Or create a small knot in the middle of the pieces already pinned back for added decoration. This style is easy to get creative with and make it uniquely yours.

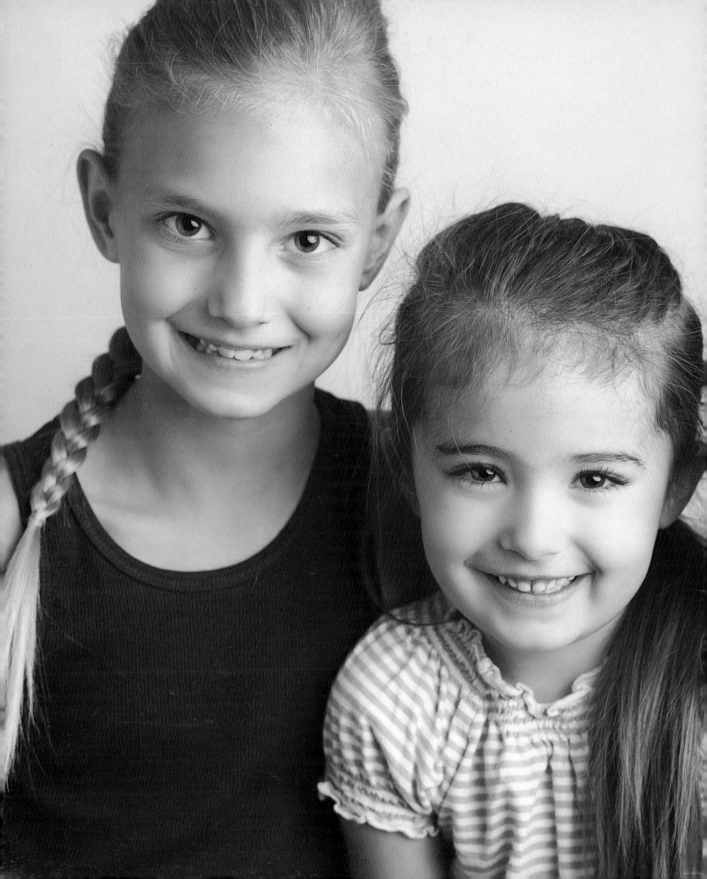

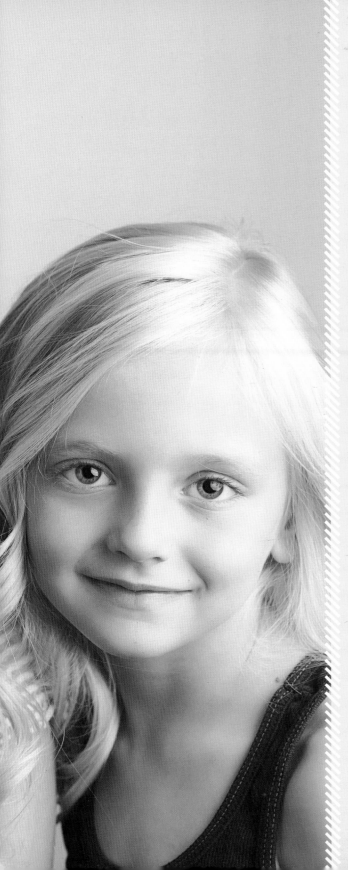

Super Styles for GIRLS

It's not just women who need a variety of looks for their locks. Little girls like to have pretty hair, too! And girls everywhere will be thanking their mothers for the fun and fresh variety of hairstyles in this section, including the essential French braids in the Double French Braid and the supercute Braided Fringe—perfect for when you need to braid those bangs your daughter has decided to grow out. I've also added a couple new styles to keep up with those creative little imaginations. Girls of all ages will get a kick out of the Twisted Sister and the Hair Bow.

The next time the daddy-daughter dance comes around, you'll have several styles available to please your little ladies. (Feel free to try them on your own hair, too!)

Hair Bow

As a mother of a little girl, I adore putting bows in my daughter's hair—anything from those small enough to fit on a barrette to very much oversize bows. This hairstyle allows you to style your little girl's hair into an actual hair bow. Your little lady will look darling with this bow atop her head. It will shine on the dance floor at a recital or add spunk to her Sunday best. Whichever way she decides to wear this bow, it's sure to be adorable. It works well with wavy and straight hairstyles.

TOOLS NEEDED

bobby pins

colorful or clear elastic bands

light-hold hairspray

teasing comb

PREPPING HER HAIR | If your child has flyaways, you can use a bit of defining paste to smooth her tresses after teasing her hair in step 2. If you like, you also can coat her ponytail with a defining paste before step 4. This helps keep those haircuts with layers all together in the hair bow.

1

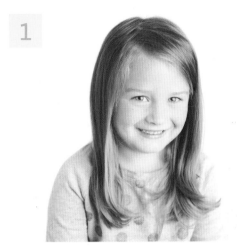

Start with dry hair.

2

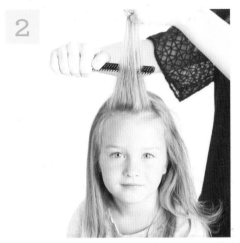

Using a teasing comb, gently tease her crown area just slightly if you prefer a little volume on top.

3

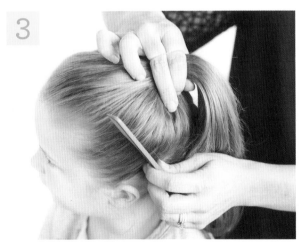

Gather her hair into a high ponytail, using a comb to smooth out any bumps along the way, and secure with a colorful elastic band.

4

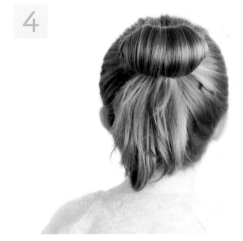

Wrap another elastic band around her ponytail, but don't pull the tail all the way through on the last pull. This creates a bun-looking top half, with the ends of her pony hanging out the bottom half.

5

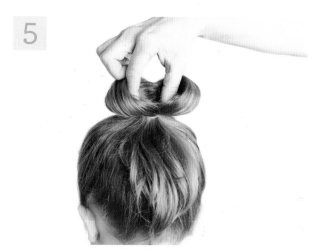

Divide the bun in two pieces down the center, creating two separate buns.

6

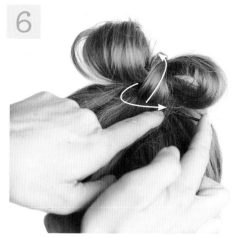

Grab a piece of hair from the ends of the ponytail that are still hanging down; wrap this piece of hair up, around, between, and over the buns; and secure with a bobby pin.

7

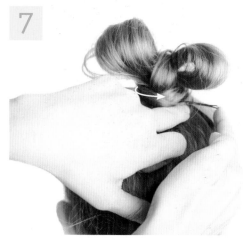

Wrap the remaining piece of hair (from the ends of the ponytail) around the base of the ponytail, and secure it with a bobby pin.

8

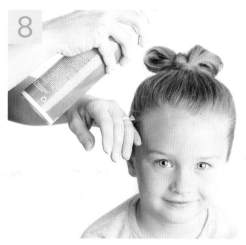

Finish with a light-hold hairspray.

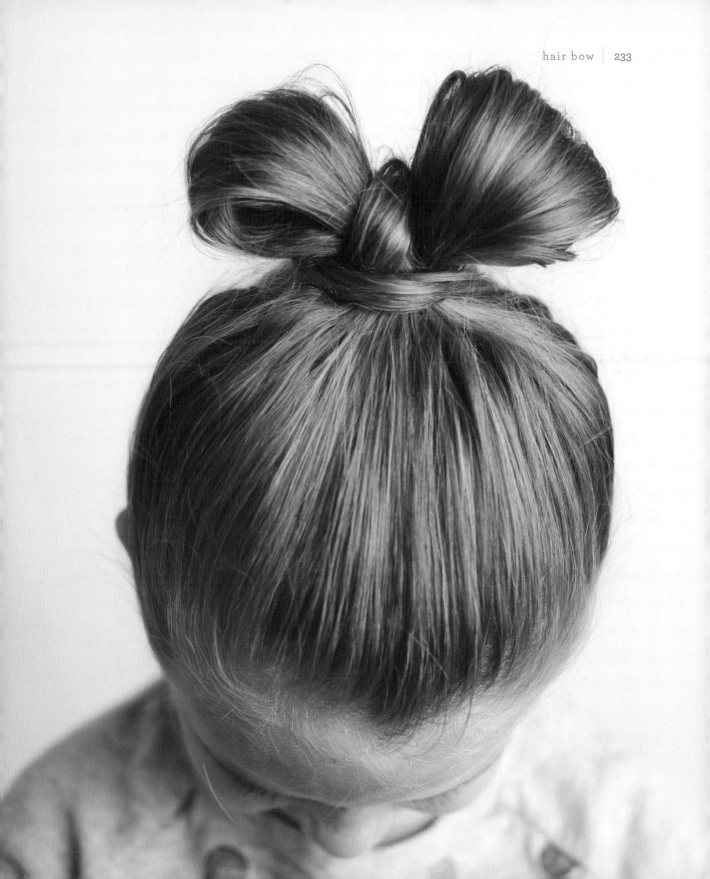

Double French Braid

The French braid is a lovely style on its own, but it's also very adaptable into other looks. This style is simply two French braids divided by a center part. It's a great way to keep hair out of your little darling's face during her next softball game or field day on her last day of school. All hair textures work well with these braids.

TOOLS NEEDED

colorful elastic bands

clips

hairspray

rattail comb

PREPPING HER HAIR | If you begin with wet hair, use a medium- to firm-hold hair gel to keep all the little hairs in place. If you begin with dry hair, dispense a dollop of defining paste about $3/4$ inch (2cm) in diameter in your palms and distribute it throughout the lengths of her hair for better grip while you're braiding.

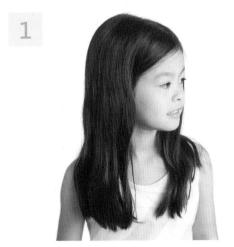

Start with her hair wet or dry.

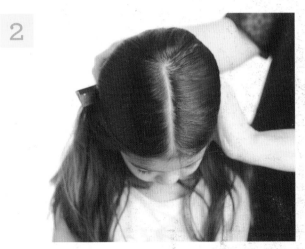

Using a rattail comb, part her hair down the center, leaving two equal sections. You can use her nose as a reference point for a perfect center part.

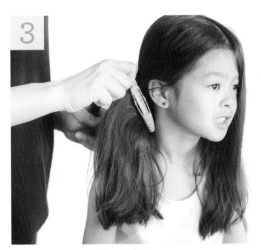

Clip one side out of the way so you can start to braid the other section.

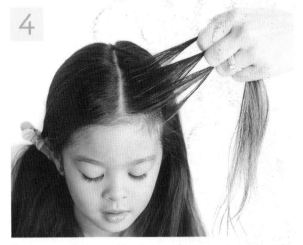

Starting on the top of her loose section, gather three pieces of hair.

5

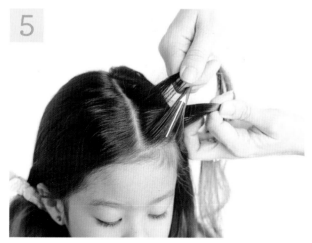

Cross the left section over the center piece.

6

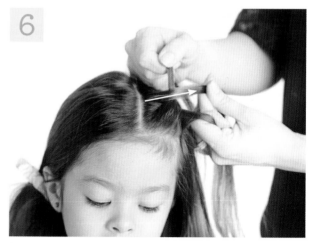

Next, cross the right section over the center piece.

7

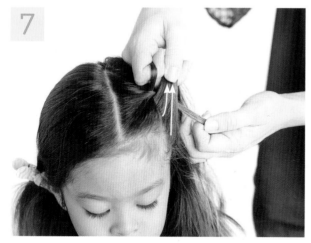

Grab a horizontal subsection of hair, and add it to the left section. Cross your newly larger left side over the center piece.

8

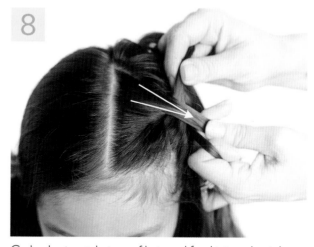

Grab a horizontal piece of hair, and feed it into the right side section. Now cross that section over the center section.

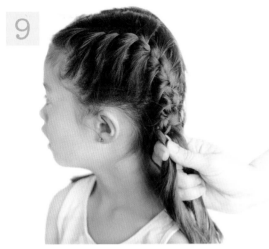

9

Continue with steps 7 and 8 until you reach the nape of her neck.

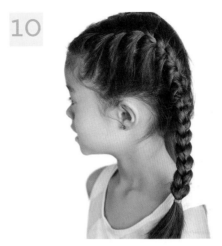

10

Continue to braid her lengths of the hair with a regular braid. Secure the ends with a colorful elastic band.

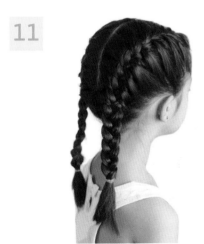

11

Unclip her hair from the other side, and braid as you did on the first side.

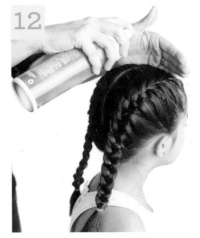

12

After you've secured the ends on the second braid, you can lightly spray with hairspray for extra hold.

If you braid your daughter's hair while it's still wet, let it dry, and take out the braids, she'll have a head full of fun and funky waves!

Twisted Sister

If you're comfortable braiding your daughter's hair using the basic braid, French braid, fishtail braid, and inside-out French braid, you may be ready for something fresh and contemporary. The Twisted Sister is a unique way to twist your girl's hair—and it's functional so she can still be a little girl with this style and not have to hold her head still all day. She can wear these ponies to brunch on Sundays or a boutique fashion show for children. Wherever she goes, she's sure to attract attention with this style. Wavy and straight hair work best with this style.

TOOLS NEEDED

colorful elastic bands
hairspray
rattail comb

PREPPING HER HAIR | You can smooth a dollop of defining paste about $7/8$ inch (2.25cm) in diameter in her hair at the very beginning before separating her hair into the ponytails for better grip and maneuvering. This also creates a more polished look if your daughter is wearing this style to a special event.

1

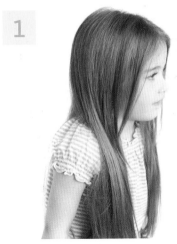

Start with dry hair that's been blown-dry and is smooth in appearance. It can have a slight wave in it, but not much.

2

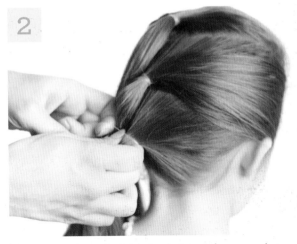

Using a rattail comb, divide her hair into three equal horizontal sections. Secure each section with a colorful elastic band so she has three separate ponytails, one on top of the other, down the back of her head.

3

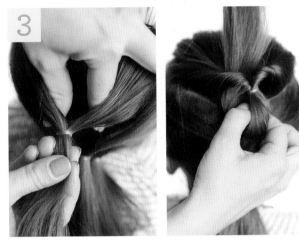

Turn the top ponytail inside out by creating a small hole directly above the first elastic band and pushing the end of the tail through the opening.

4

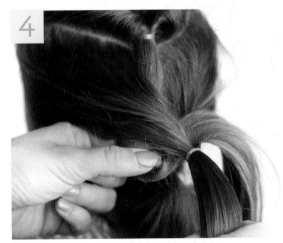

Create an opening in the second ponytail (the middle one), and pull the tail of the *top* ponytail through the hole in the second.

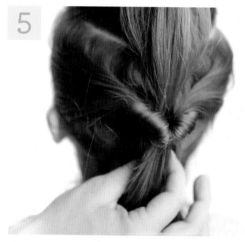

After you've pulled the tail is through, create a new opening in the second ponytail just above the elastic band, and pull the ponytail over and through the opening.

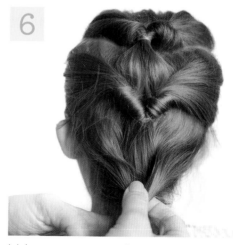

Make an opening just above the elastic band in the third, bottom ponytail. Pull the tail from the *second* pony through the bottom opening. After you pull the ponytail through, you can use an additional elastic band to secure it.

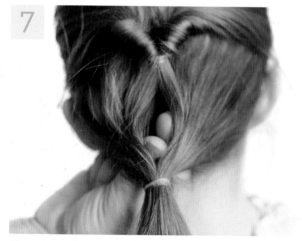

Create yet another opening directly above the elastic band, and pull the end of the third ponytail over and into the opening, pulling the ponytail all the way through.

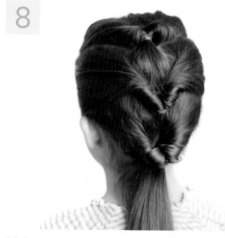

All three inside-out ponies should be connected now.

9

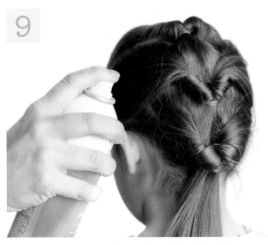

Finish with hairspray for additional hold and to smooth hairs around the hairline

For a bit of volume on the top of her head, you can tease her crown with a teasing comb before separating it into ponytails.

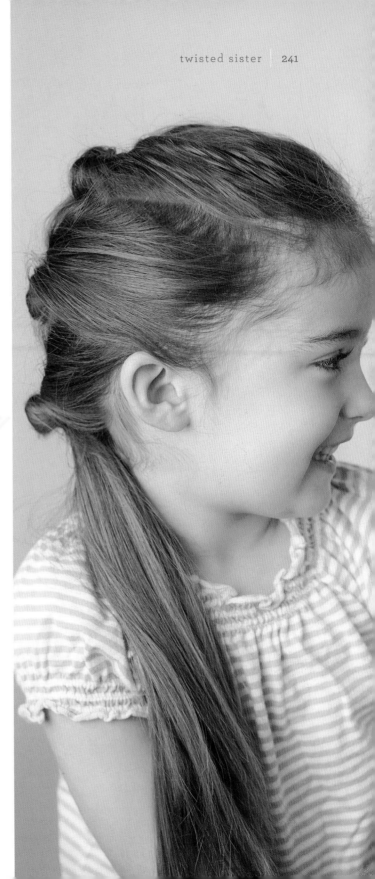

Braided Fringe

This style is great if your daughter is growing out her fringe, or bangs. You can use clips and headbands to corral her bangs while they're growing, but the Braided Fringe gives her hair a bit more style while it keeps those stray hairs in check. You also could implement this style before pulling her hair into a ponytail for sporting events or before going swimming. All hair types and textures work with this style; her bangs need to be longer than 2 inches (5cm) long though.

TOOLS NEEDED

- clear elastic bands
- clips
- hairspray
- rattail comb

PREPPING HER HAIR | If her hair is wet, apply a gel for control. If it's dry, use a defining paste. Whichever product you use, disperse a pea-size amount throughout her bangs.

1

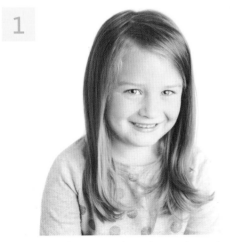

Her hair can be wet or dry to begin this style.

2

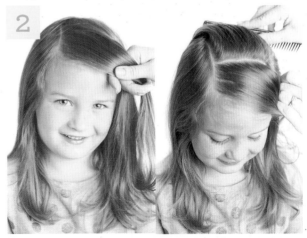

Using a rattail comb and the arch of her eyebrow as a guide, begin parting her hair for the braid. The part should be approximately 1 or 2 inches (2.5 to 5cm) back from her hairline and can go across and down her head as far as you like.

3

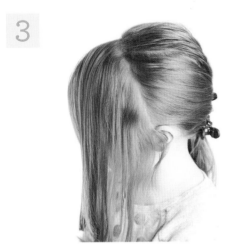

Clip all her remaining hair out of the way, leaving the parted section down and ready to braid.

4

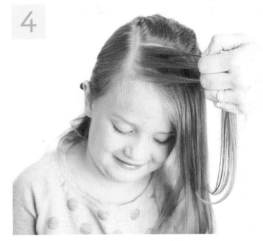

Starting at the top far section, closest to the center of her head, gather a smaller subsection and divide it into three separate sections.

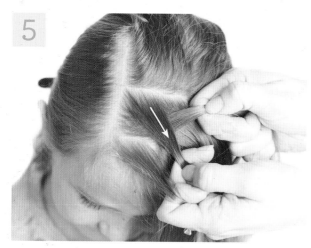

Cross the right section over the center section.

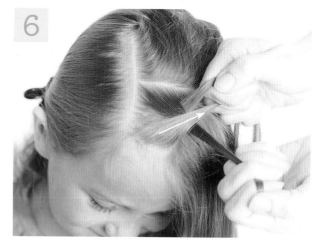

Then cross the left section over the center section.

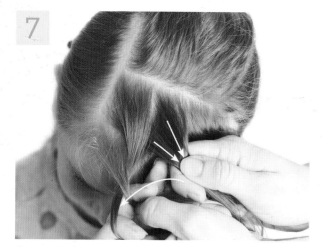

Grab a small subsection from the right side and add it into the right subsection. Cross that piece of hair over the center section.

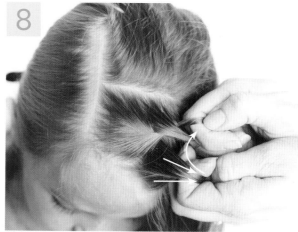

Grab a horizontal subsection of hair from the left side and add it into the left subsection. Cross the left piece of hair over the center subsection.

9

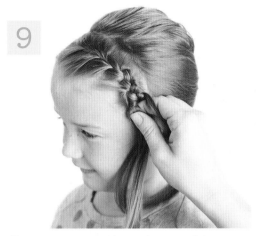

Continue steps 7 and 8 until you reach her ear, or wherever you'd like to stop the braid.

10

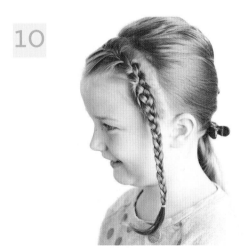

Secure the braid with a colorful elastic band, or continue braiding her hair using a regular braid until you reach the ends and then secure with an elastic band. Spray with hairspray for hold.

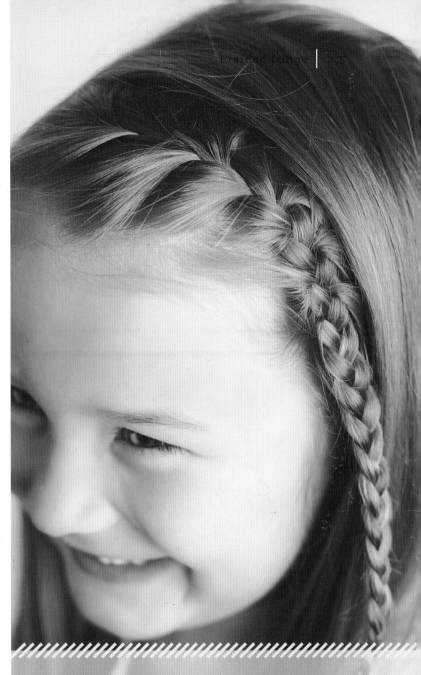

If you want to pull her hair into a ponytail after braiding her bangs, you can curl the ends of her hair for a more formal look before putting it into a ponytail. If you're using the braid more for function instead of fashion, you can leave the strands in their natural form before putting her hair into a ponytail.

Inside-Out French Braid

The French braid is a classic and great for pulling active girls' hair up in a chic way. And she'll love this inside-out twist on the basic French braid. She can wear this look to her ballet class, the trampoline park, or a fun day at the zoo. No matter where this style takes her, she'll look terrific. All hair types and textures work with this fun style.

TOOLS NEEDED

clear elastic bands
hairspray
rattail comb

PREPPING HER HAIR | Before you begin

braiding her hair, you can add a dollop of defining paste about 7/8 inch (2.25cm) in diameter to your palms and run it through the lengths of her hair to tame it and fight frizz.

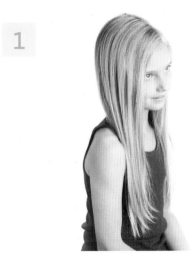

Start with dry hair.

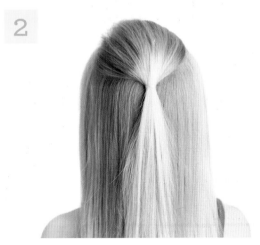

Gather a small section of hair in her crown area. You can use a rattail comb to define this section of hair if you like. Secure it with a clear elastic band, and let the ponytail hang down the back of her head.

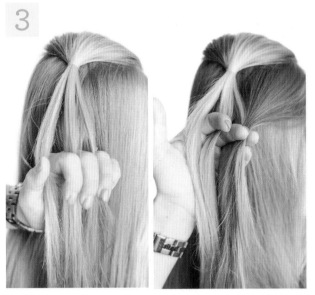

Divide the small ponytail into three subsections. Grab a small horizontal section of hair below her ponytail on the right side, and add it to the right subsection.

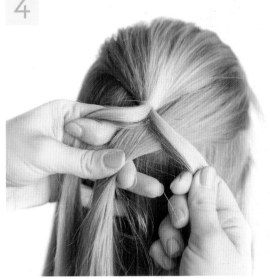

Slide that right section *underneath* the center subsection. (The previous right section is now the center section.)

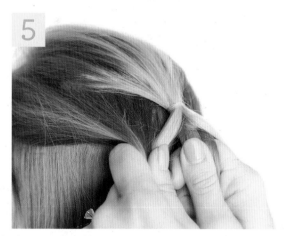

Gather a horizontal subsection just beneath her ponytail on the left side of her head, and add that section to the left subsection.

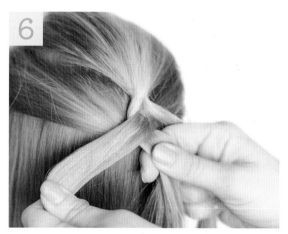

Weave the left section underneath the center subsection. (The previous subsection on the left is now the center section.)

Note that unlike a regular French braid, where you'd cross the sections *over* each other, in this inside-out version, you slide the sections *under* each other. This is key to achieving that inside-out look.

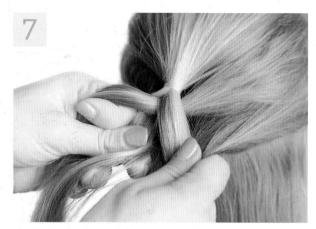

Gather the next horizontal section of hair, add it to the right subsection, and slide that section under the center subsection.

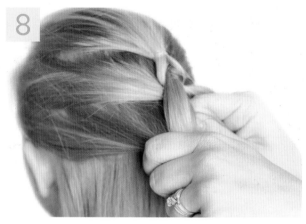

Gather the next horizontal piece of hair from the left side of her head, add it into the left subsection, and weave that under the center subsection.

9

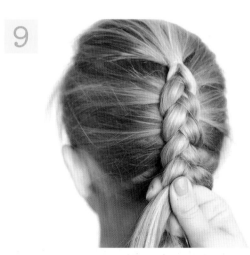

Continue down her head, repeating steps 7 and 8, until you reach the nape of her neck.

10

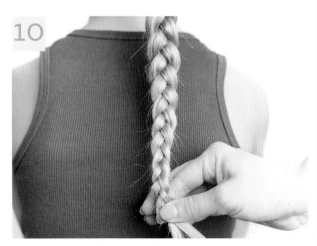

When you reach the nape of her neck, continue weaving her hair in a backward motion until you reach the ends, and secure with an elastic band. You can finish with hairspray to tame flyaways and keep the hairstyle intact.

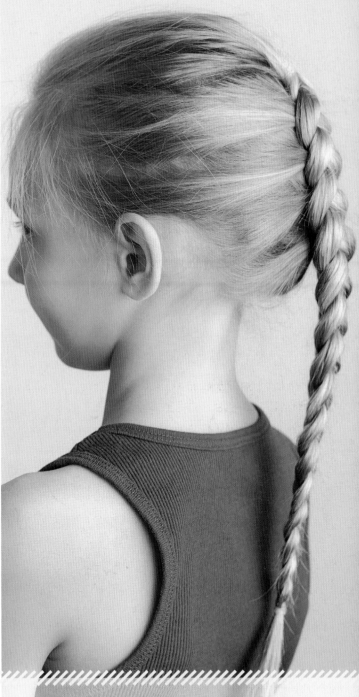

If you don't want it to show, you can cut and remove the elastic band at the top of the braid, or you can cover it with pieces of hair from the top of her braid.

Glossary

all-purpose comb   This general comb has many uses, hence the name. It's best to have one that's heat resistant so you can use it to guide and keep your hair smooth while you use heat-producing styling tools. A good general comb can also be used to mold hair into up-dos.

antifrizz serum   A product that combats frizz by surrounding your hair strands with a protective, moisturizing coating. Depending on the type of serum, it can be used wet or dry and works best to combat frizz and tame unruly hair. In some cases, it can even reduce the time your hair takes to dry.

antihumectant serum   A styling product that blocks moisture, prevents frizz, and can help smooth your hair and tame flyaways.

argan oil   This oil, produced from kernels from a tree grown in Morocco, contains vitamins and essential fatty acids beneficial for your hair. It's ideal if your hair is in distress or needs moisture. As it absorbs into your hair, it hydrates and repairs. It can be used on wet or dry locks.

blow-dryer   This indispensable tool blows hot air or cool air at various speeds. A blow-dryer's main purpose is to dry wet hair, but you also can use it to help form your hair into a specific style, such as a blowout.

blowout   A hairstyle created by applying a product to damp hair and then blowing-dry the hair using a paddle brush and round brush for a voluminous effect. All lengths of hair can achieve this style in different variations.

boar bristle brush   A brush that polishes your hair as you brush, thanks to the natural boar bristles that help distribute your hair's natural oils.

bob   A short hairstyle; the length hits right at the jawline. The bob was especially popular in the 1920s.

bobby pin   A styling aid that helps hold your hairstyle in place. Bobby pins are an especially essential part of an up-do style. Most standard-size bobby pins are about 2 or 3 inches (5 to 7.5cm) long. (Larger and smaller sizes are also sold.) They come in a variety of colors to blend in to many hair colors.

chignon   A French word that means "nape of the neck." Also, a hairstyle in which a low-slung bun or knot sits close to the nape of the neck. These are usually worn in a formal setting and typically have a smooth and polished appearance.

clear elastic band   *See* elastic band.

clip   Many sizes, shapes, and types of hair clips are available, but most often in this book, *clip* refers to a sturdy pinching clip with grips on one side to hold hair in place. You can find these clips at your beauty supply store.

concentrator   This device fits on the end of a blow-dryer and concentrates and directs air and heat flow through so you can dry your hair smoothly. Using a concentrator on your blow-dryer means you can get smoother and more polished hair without the use of a straightening iron.

cowlick   A section of hair that misbehaves. It could fall differently from the rest of the hair around it or stand straight up.

crimping iron   A version of a curling or flatting iron that's designed kink your hair into sharp, chevron or zigzag waves. This look was popular in the 1980s but is making a comeback on runways and costume parties everywhere.

crown   The top of the head. The hair in this area is easy to tease to create volume.

curl cream   This multipurpose product defines your curls while also providing a light hold—without weighing down your locks like other products can do. You can layer curl cream with a light- or firm-hold gel for maximum hold in your style. It is best applied to damp hair and then left to air dry or blow-dry with a diffuser.

curling iron   A curling iron is a handheld tool with a barrel on one end that heats up. You coil your hair around the hot barrel, close the clamp to keep your hair against the barrel, hold for a few seconds, and unclamp for curly locks. Multiple barrel sizes are available, ranging from $3/8$ inch (1cm) to 2 inches (5cm). The larger the barrel, the larger your curls.

curling wand   A handheld styling tool similar to a curling iron but without a clamp to hold your hair. This heated rod is great for getting mermaid waves.

defining paste   This is a lightweight finishing product can be used to softly mold your hair. Shorter hairstyles can really reap the benefits of this paste; applying a small amount throughout your hair adds texture.

diffuser   This attachment fits on the end of your blow-dryer and is designed to enhance your curls by diffusing the air and heat widely and evenly. It also reduces frizz when drying curly hair.

dry conditioner   You can use this product to hydrate your hair from the middle of your strands to the ends; it absorbs oil as it works. Some contain sunflower oil or argan oil for additional moisture.

dry shampoo   This shampoo is every girl's best friend and a quick-and-easy hairstyle extender. By using this oil-absorber, you can get away with a 2- or 3-day-old style. You also can add texture to your hair by applying dry shampoo to your roots and teasing with a teasing comb. This is great for formal styles as well.

duckbill clip   This silver metal clip is approximately 2½ inches (5cm) long and has two prongs. The duckbill clip is commonly used to hold and set curls after they've been curled with a curling iron. *See also* clip.

elastic band   The clear version of these rubber bands, often no larger than ½ to ¾ inch (1.25 to 2cm) in diameter, are commonly used in up-styles and formal hairdos. Because they're clear, they camouflage into your hair, so no one but you knows they're there. Colored elastic bands are also available—perfect for little girls. These add a pop of color to the end of a braid or around ponytails.

fabric hairband   A modern, decorative version of a hair tie for when you want a quick and easy splash of color in your hair. Emi-Jay is one brand.

firm-hold gel   This gel is built to set your hair with maximum hold. You might see formal styles and up-dos call for this product before blow-drying to ensure the style lasts all night. If you have curly hair that's somewhat defiant, you might try using this gel for some better control.

fishtail braid   A variation of a braid that's woven to look like a fishbone.

flat iron   A flat iron, or straightening iron, is another handheld tool that uses heat to style your hair. This tool has two ceramic plates that close together, sandwiching your hair in between, to smooth and flatten your hair. Flat irons can get extremely hot, reaching temperatures upward of 400°F (205°C).

French braid   A braid that starts at the top of the head and is woven downward to the very ends of the hair.

fringe   Another term for bangs. It's the area typically from the edge of one eyebrow to the other on the front hairline.

hair-dryer   *See* blow-dryer.

hairpin   A U-shape pin, similar to a bobby pin, that secures your locks without disrupting the flow of your hairstyle. Whereas a bobby pin offers firm hold, hairpins have a very loose and natural hold. This is due to their design—both legs of hairpins are smooth, and they're separated a bit more than the legs of bobby pins. Hairpins also come in different lengths and colors.

hairline   The area where your hair meets your skin.

heat-resistant comb   A comb that can stand up to the heat produced by hot tools and won't melt. These are important to have when using hot tools.

hot roller   Cylindrical curling tools that heat up in an electric device. When they're hot, you put them into your hair and clip them into place to allow your curls to set. When they're cool, you remove them and your hair will be curly.

hydrating conditioner If you have a curly coif or are prone to frizz, this is the conditioner for you. A hydrating conditioner containing aloe or olive oil can naturally help your hair revive itself. Use a hydrating conditioner during the dry winter months to ward off static.

hydrating shampoo This cleanser is normally a bit heavier and made for dry or dull hair. If you have fine hair, you'll most likely want to avoid hydrating or moisturizing shampoos because they could weigh down your hair. Medium to thick and coarse hair types benefit most from this cleanser.

iron guard spray A spray that helps protect your hair from hot styling tools. Typically this spray is used on dry hair; you can use some protectant sprays on wet hair as well.

leave-in conditioner This conditioner comes in either a cream or a spray. Most leave-in treatments contain a moisture-retention ingredient as well as something to help protect your hair. In addition, these revitalizers can come in different levels of moisture depending on your hair type. Most also help with shine.

long metal clip This long, flat, and metal clip ranges from 2 to 4 inches (5 to 10cm) long. This type of clip is commonly used to hold curls or mold hairstyles without leaving any creases like a duckbill clip might. *See also* clip.

maximum-hold hairspray This hairspray usually includes an antihumectant ingredient that protects your hair from the environment to prolong your style. Some can feel stiff when in your hair; however, other modern, heavy-hold sprays contain lighter ingredients that won't weigh down your hair. Max-hold sprays are typically used in formal styles or ones you don't want to move … at all.

moisturizing serum This product—be it argan oil, an antifrizz serum, or any kind of serum that contains moisturizing ingredients—is used to soften and relax hair.

molding paste *See* defining paste.

mousse Also known as styling foam, this multitasking product can be used to add volume not only to your roots, but also to the ends of your hair while providing a light hold. It tames and forms your hair but doesn't leave it crunchy and dry.

paddle brush This large, flat brush is used to detangle and help reduce drying time when blow-drying. The bristles are designed to be gentle on wet and dry strands. It can even give you a slight scalp massage when you brush through your hair thoroughly.

part A division in your hair. You create a part by drawing a line on your scalp with a comb or your fingers.

pomade This light-hold finishing product defines your strands and adds polish and shine.

pompadour   A short hairstyle that was made popular in the 1950s. In this style, the hair is teased in the front and smoothed back to blend. This hairstyle has made a comeback with modern adaptations.

rattail comb   This comb has small teeth on one end and a straight, pointy pick on the other end. The pointy end is helpful for precisely sectioning and parting your hair before styling.

recession point   Your recession points are located at the top corners of your front hairline, just above the outer corners of your eyebrows.

repairing conditioner   This rejuvenating product often contains a type of protein or keratin treatment to help strengthen weak or damaged hair. If you frequently color your hair or use hot tools in it regularly, you should use this type of conditioner at least once a week.

repairing shampoo   This shampoo shifts your hair into repair mode after your mane has been abused with heat or harsh chemicals. It also helps reduce breakage.

roller   A cylindrical curling tool that, when heated, can curl your hair. *See also* hot roller.

root   The area where your hair comes out of your scalp.

root lifter   This root booster gives you lift at the root of your hair or in your crown area. Opt for a root lifter that's not full of stickiness but one that leaves your hair soft and touchable.

round brush   This brush will soon become your favorite. It's essential for smoothing, taming, and curling your hair. Opt for a vented version if you can find one. Many sizes of round brushes are available to yield different styles. A smaller round brush produces a curly or wavier look on the middle and ends of your hair. A larger size mainly smooths your hair and adds a slight bend at the ends.

sculpting lotion   This light-hold gel formula gives hair hold without weighing it down. It's best to use before you curl your hair or to add longevity to your style.

sea-salt spray   This blend, which you typically spray on the ends of your hair, assists in creating a natural wave look. Those with naturally wavy or curly hair can achieve soft waves by using this mist; straight strands can get texture and a touch of bend.

shine spray   Used mostly as a finishing product, this mist is designed to enhance shine and bring life to dull hair. If you don't wash your hair every day, using this spray in addition to the dry conditioner could revive the ends of your hair. You also might like using this spray before you gently comb through your curls.

smoothing serum   This product, which could be considered a moisturizing serum, typically contains an antifrizz or antihumectant property to coax wavy, coarse, or curly hair smooth and straight. Many also now contain protectants to help prevent future damage.

sock bun sponge This styling aid helps you form the perfect bun. These doughnut-shape sponges enable you to pull your ponytail through the center hole and then pin your hair around the doughnut to create a full, round bun. If you have trouble forming a voluminous bun with just your hair alone, try a sock bun sponge. They're available in different colors and sizes.

split end A condition in which the ends of your strand of hair are literally split in two. This is a sign your hair has some damage and is in need of a trim.

spray wax A new delivery of an old favorite, this wax has a light to medium hold that's meant to add a touch of texture and grit to hair. Fine to medium hair types will benefit from this tress plumper.

stretchy ponytail holder A large, stretchy band that contains a coating over the elastic or rubber band so it doesn't pull or break your hair when you're putting it in or taking it out. These bands come in different sizes to suit a variety of hair thickness. They're great for securing ponytails for maximum hold if the clear elastic isn't strong enough.

styling foam Also known as mousse, this multitasking product can be used to add volume not only to your roots but also to the ends of your hair while providing a light hold. It tames and forms your hair but doesn't leave it crunchy and dry.

teasing brush A brush that usually contains nylon and boar bristles that's designed to add volume or texture to your hair.

teasing comb This comb contains three rows of teeth and is used to backcomb your hair to create more volume. Don't use just any comb to tease your hair; a teasing comb is vital for creating volume without damaging your hair.

texture putty Similar to defining paste, this putty gives you a strong yet workable hold. Texture putty works best for shaping shorter styles. Many are transparent and can be used on all hair types, but if the putty is light in color, it's best to use it on lighter-colored hair.

texturizing spray A styling product that adds more movement or grit to your original hair texture. Spray wax or sea-salt spray are examples.

thermal protectant If you frequently use hot tools, you also should frequently use this product. Thermal protectant is normally sold as a spray or cream and contains essential oils to hydrate your hair. In addition, it helps protect your hair from humidity and contains beneficial antioxidants and proteins.

thickening conditioner This conditioner is meant to be used alongside thickening shampoo and adds natural volume to limp or lifeless stands. This booster softens and separates your strands without weighing them down.

thickening lotion This plumper, designed to cover each of your strands to make them fuller, is best for very fine hair that needs more body. It can double as a light-hold product as well.

thickening shampoo   This shampoo is best for those whose hair is thinning or who have very fine hair to begin with. It normally contains an exfoliating ingredient to give your strands the best possible foundation for growth. Half of the reason hair doesn't grow—other than genetics—is follicle asphyxiation, meaning your follicles are smothered and, therefore, stop growing. The thickening shampoo helps clear away what's smothering your follicles so your hair can grow again.

three-barrel curling iron   A curling iron that has three barrels—typically two on the bottom and one on the top. Pressing your hair between the barrels creates soft, uniform waves.

vent brush   A brush with slots, or vents, cut in the body of the brush, between the bristles. When you use a vent brush as you blow-dry your hair, air flows through these vents and around your hair, enabling you to dry it faster.

volumizing conditioner   This weightless formula is meant to soften your tresses without leaving behind any residue that might weigh down your 'do. Fine to medium hair types benefit from a lightweight cream conditioner.

volumizing hairspray   A hairspray that promotes volume with a firm hold. It usually has stronger hold to help hold and amplify hair for a voluminous look.

volumizing powder   Sprinkle this fairy dust–looking product on your roots for added fullness. Some even reactivate throughout the day with a little heat and friction from your fingers. This gives you a tousled, voluminous look.

volumizing shampoo   This lightweight shampoo is meant to give limp locks some lift. It's usually (or should be) clear in color and should give your hair a weightless feel. This purifier shouldn't strip your hair of its natural oils.

water bottle   A spray water bottle you can use to wet your hair when you need moisture during a style. You can find these at your local drug store or beauty supply store.

wide-tooth comb   The teeth on this comb are spaced a bit wider apart than on other types of combs. This helps you gently work through tangles.

working hairspray   A working hairspray is brushable and provides moveable hold. This spray should be heavy enough to hold the style, but not give you a stiff look or feel. More recently, lighter-weight working hairsprays are dry. The dry sprays provide hold without the stickiness that often accompanies wet sprays.

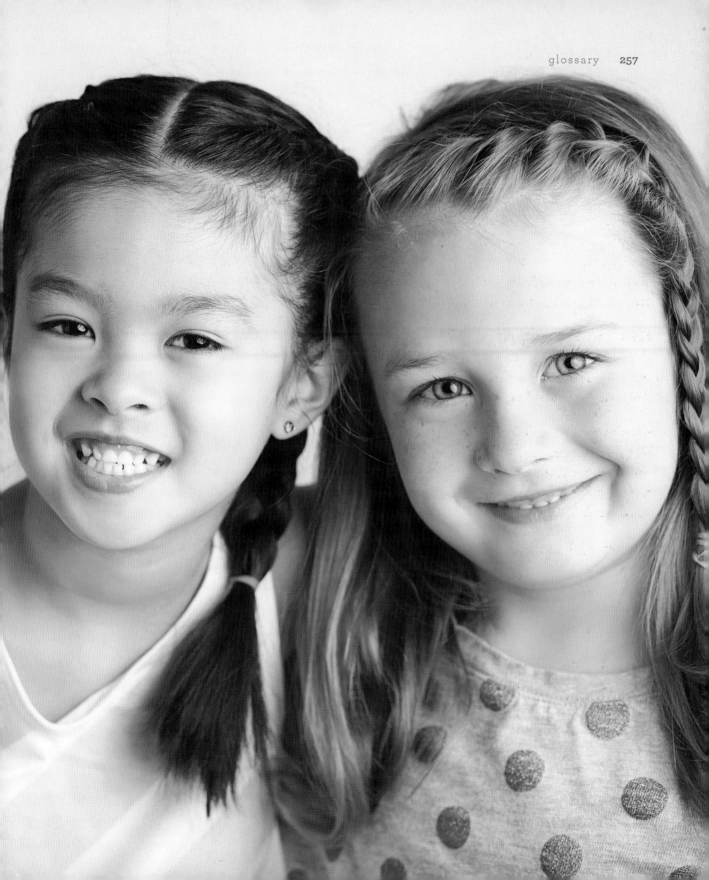

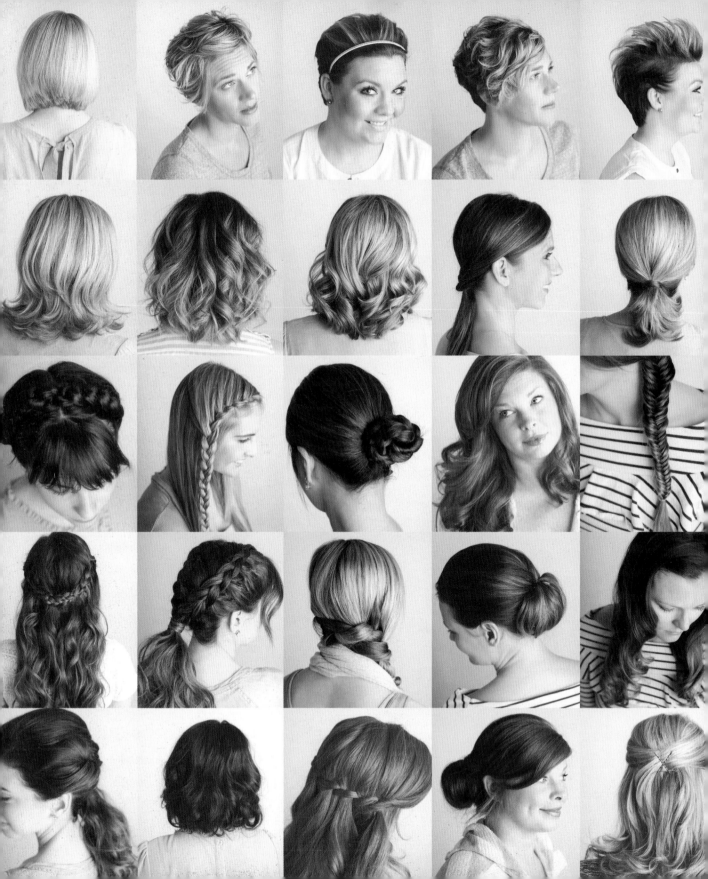

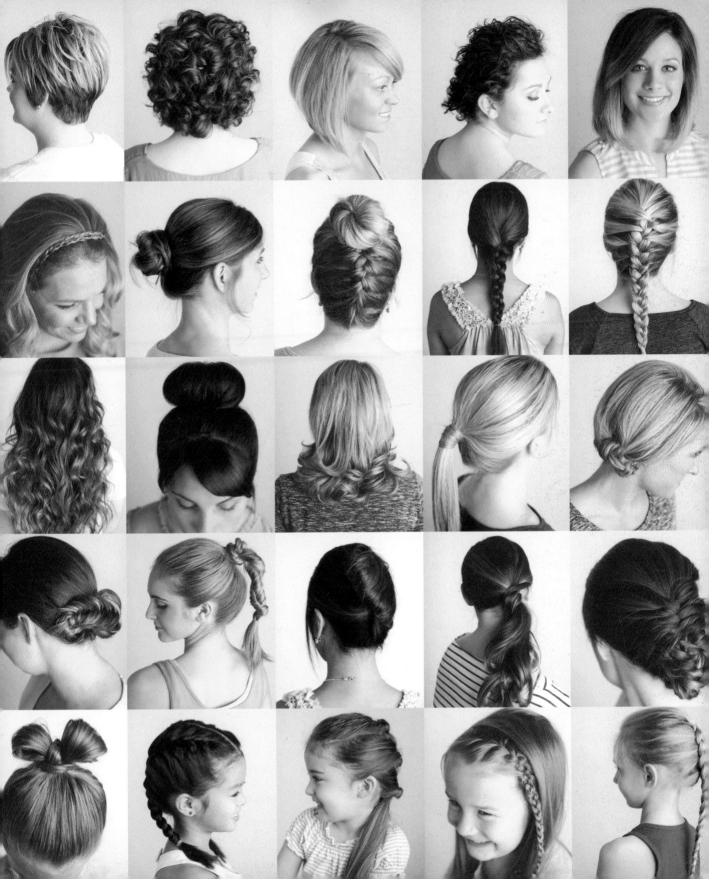

Index

A

all-purpose comb, 12
antifrizz serum, 8
antihumectant serum, 8
argan oil, 8

B

bangs
    Short Hair Blowout, 36
    Sleek and Straight, 29
    Twisted, 32
Basic Blowout, 66–69
Basic Braid, 104–107
Beach Waves, 74–77
Bear Claw Ponytail, 164–167
blow-dryer, 10
    fragile hair and, 22
blowout
    medium-length hair, 66–69
    short hair, 34-37
bobby pins, 14
Bombshell Curls, 130–133
Braided Bun, 122–125
Braided Fringe, 242–245
Braided Headband, 90–93
braids
    Basic Braid, 104–107
    Braided Bun, 122–125
    Braided Fringe, 242–245
    Broken Fishbone, 199–201
    Crown and Glory, 154–157
    Double French Braid, 234–237
    Festival Braided Knot, 158–163
    Fishtail, 126–129
    Fishtail Bun, 178–183
    Inchworm Braid, 118–121
    Inside-Out French Braid, 246–249
    Prairie Braid, 112–117
    Upside-Down Braided Knot, 98–101
    Waterfall Braid, 214–217
Broken Fishbone, 199–201
brushes/combs, 12
buns
    Braided Bun, 122–125
    Fishtail Bun, 178–183
    Knot Your Basic Bun, 150–153
    Side Bun, 218–223
    Simple Chignon, 170–173
    sock bun sponges, 15
    Undone Bun, 82–85

C

clips, 14
combs/brushes, 12
concentrator (blow-dryer), 10
conditioner, 5
crimping irons, 10
Crown and Glory, 154–157
curls
    Bombshell Curls, 130–133
    curl cream, 6

curling iron, 10
curling wands, 10
Curly Girl, 50–53

D–E

defining paste, 9
diffuser (blow-dryer), 10
Double French Braid, 234–237
dry conditioner, 5
dry shampoo, 5
duckbill clips, 14

elastic bands, 15

F

Faux Bob, 208–213
Festival Braided Knot, 158–163
fine hair
    frizz taming, 20
    volume, 18
firm-hold gel, 6
Fishtail, 126–129
Fishtail Bun, 178–183
flat iron, 10
Flipped Out, 70–73
French Braid, 108–111
French Twist, 190–193
frizz taming, 20–21

G

girls' styles, 229
    Braided Fringe, 242–245
    Double French Braid, 234–237
    Hair Bow, 230–233
    Inside-Out French Braid, 246–249
    Twisted Sister, 238–341

H

hairbands, 15
    Braided Headband, 90
Hair Bow, 230–233
hairpins, 14
hairspray
    maximum-hold, 8
    volumizing, 8
    working, 8
Half Twist, 202–207
Half Up, 224–227
High Roller, 142–145
hydrating conditioner, 5
hydrating shampoo, 5

I–J–K

Inchworm Braid, 118–121
Inside-Out French Braid, 246–249
Inside-Out Pony, 94–97

Knot Your Basic Bun, 150–153

L

leave-in conditioner, 5
long hair styles, 103
  Basic Braid, 104–107
  Bear Claw Ponytail, 164–167
  Bombshell Curls, 130–133
  Braided Bun, 122–125
  Crown and Glory, 154–157
  Festival Braided Knot, 158–163
  Fishtail, 126–129
  French Braid, 108–111
  High Roller, 142–145
  Inchworm Braid, 118–121
  Knot Your Basic Bun, 150–153
  Mermaid Waves, 135–137
  Polished Pony, 146–149
  Prairie Braid, 112–117
  Top Knot, 138–141
long metal clips, 15

M–N–O

maximum-hold hairspray, 8
medium-length hair styles, 65
  Basic Blowout, 66–69
  Beach Waves, 74–77
  Braided Headband, 90–93
  Flipped Out, 70–73
  Inside-Out Pony, 94–97
  Party Pony, 86–89
  Polished Coils, 78–81
  Undone Bun, 82–85
  Upside-Down Braided Knot, 98–101

medium-thick hair
  frizz taming, 20
  volume, 18
Mermaid Waves, 135–137
moisturizing serum, 8

P-Q

paddle brush, 12
Party Pony, 86–89
Polished Coils, 78–81
Polished Pompadour, 42–45
Polished Pony, 146–149
pomade, 9
pompadour, 42–45
ponytail holders, 15
ponytails
  Bear Claw Ponytail, 164–167
  Inside-out Pony, 94–97
  Party Pony, 86–89
  Polished Pony, 146–149
  Short and Sassy Pony, 58–63
  Side-Swept Pony, 194–197
  Twisted Pony, 184–189
Prairie Braid, 112–117

R

rattail comb, 12
repairing conditioner, 5
repairing shampoo, 5
Retro Waves, 174–177
root lifter, 6
round brush, 12

S

sculpting lotion, 6
sea-salt spray, 8
shampoo, 4–5
shine spray, 8
shiny hair, 22–23
Short and Sassy Pony, 58–63
Short Hair Blowout, 34–37
short hair styling, 25
    Curly Girl, 50–53
    Polished Pompadour, 42–45
    Short and Sassy Pony, 58–63
    Short Hair Blowout, 34–37
    Side Swept, 54–57
    Sleek and Straight, 26–29
    Sleek Look, 46–49
    Tousled Texture, 38–41
    Twisted, 30–32
Side Bun, 218–223
Side Swept, 54–57
Side-Swept Pony, 194–197
Simple Chignon, 170–173
Sleek and Straight, 26–29
Sleek Look, 46–49
smoothing serum, 9
sock bun sponges, 15
special occasion styles, 169
    Broken Fishbone, 199–201
    Faux Bob, 208–213
    Fishtail Bun, 178–183
    French Twist, 190–193
    Half Twist, 202–207
    Half Up, 224–227
    Retro Waves, 174–177
    Side Bun, 218–223
    Side-Swept Pony, 194–197
    Simple Chignon, 170–173
    Twisted Pony, 184–189
    Waterfall Braid, 214–217
spray wax, 9
styling aids, 14–15
styling foam, 6
styling products, 6

T

teasing comb/brush, 13
texture putty, 9
thermal protectant, 9
thick hair
    frizz taming, 20
    volume, 18
thickening conditioner, 5
thickening lotion, 6
thickening shampoo, 4
tools/equipment, 10–13
Top Knot, 138–141
Tousled Texture, 38–41
Twisted, 30–32
Twisted Pony, 184–189
Twisted Sister, 238–341

U

Undone Bun, 82–85
Upside-Down Braided Knot, 98–101

V

vent brushes, 13
volume, 18–19
    volumizing conditioner, 5
    volumizing hairspray, 8
    volumizing powder, 6
    volumizing shampoo, 4

W-X-Y-Z

Waterfall Braid, 214–217
wavy hair
    Retro Waves, 174–177
wide-tooth comb, 13
working hairspray, 8